Simulation Scenarios
for Nurse Educators

Suzanne Hetzel Campbell, PhD, WHNP-BC, IBCLC, graduated with her BS and MS in Nursing from the University of Connecticut, and her PhD in Nursing from the University of Rhode Island. She obtained her post-master's certificate as a Women's Health Nurse Practitioner from Boston College. Presently, she is Associate Professor, Associate Dean for Academic Programs, and Project Director for the Fairfield University School of Nursing Robin Kanarek Learning Resource Center. She has been teaching at Fairfield University since 2000. Her increasing interest in web-enhanced learning and simulation-based pedagogy has led to publications and workshops on these topics using her own experience to empower nursing faculty. Suzanne has been Board member and faculty liaison for the School of Nursing Advisory Board for the past three years. She is overseeing a $1.06 million-dollar four-year project which has included building renovation, classroom upgrades, faculty development, and integration of simulation throughout the nursing curriculum. The project includes a five-year assessment plan which will examine program, faculty, and student outcomes in relationship to the integration of simulation and other technology. In addition, Suzanne is certified as an International Board Certified Lactation Consultant (IBCLC), she is the country coordinator for Ireland for Fairfield University School of Nursing and serves as Director-at-Large to the Board of the International Lactation Consultant Association (ILCA) (Term 2006–2009).

Karen M. Daley, PhD, RN, graduated from Villanova University with her BSN, from Troy State University with a MS in Nursing, and a PhD in Nursing from Rutgers, the State University of New Jersey. Presently, she is Associate Professor and Graduate Nursing Coordinator for the Department of Nursing at Western Connecticut State University. Her academic interests currently involve assessment of outcomes in nursing programs through standardized testing, fostering collegiality and caring between faculty and students, and integrating simulation in nursing education. At Western Connecticut State University, Karen has spearheaded the implementation of human patient simulation throughout the curriculum and is primarily responsible for the acquisition of SimMan technology, the expansion and development of the Nursing Labs and the Nursing Resource Center, and the upgrade of resources for the Nursing Labs. As the chair of the Learning Resources Committee, Karen was able to acquire additional lab space for an additional SimMan Lab, an Assessment Lab, a technology classroom, and a Ped/OB area. A new ICU lab opened in the fall of 2008 funded by a federal nursing initiative. Karen continues to work to upgrade and integrate simulation into the nursing curriculum, train faculty in simulation-focused learning experiences in their classes, and encourage the use of simulation.

Simulation Scenarios for Nurse Educators

Making It Real

Suzanne Hetzel Campbell, PhD, WHNP-BC, IBCLC
■ Karen M. Daley, PhD, RN ■ Editors

SPRINGER PUBLISHING COMPANY
New York

Springer Publishing Company, LLC
11 West 42nd Street
New York, NY 10036–8002
www.springerpub.com

Acquisitions Editor: Allan Graubard
Project Manager: Wendy Druck
Cover Design: David Levy
Composition: Aptara, Inc.

09 10 11 12 13/   5 4 3 2 1

Ebook ISBN: 978-08261-22438

_____

Library of Congress Cataloging-in-Publication Data

Campbell, Suzanne Hetzel.
   Simulation scenarios for nurse educators : making it real / Suzanne Hetzel Campbell, Karen M. Daley.
       p. ; cm.
Includes bibliographical references and index.
ISBN 978-0-8261-2242-1
1. Nursing – Study and teaching – Simulation methods. 2. Simulated patients.
I. Daley, Karen M. II. Title.
[DNLM: 1. Education, Nursing – methods. 2. Patient Simulation. 3. Curriculum.
4. Education, Nursing – trends. WY 18.8 C191s 2009]
RT73.C27   2009
610.7307–dc22   2008038337

_____

Printed in Canada by Transcontinental Printing

This book is dedicated to all those who have helped along the way. To our husbands and families who never stop believing, supporting, and inspiring us: You are the wings upon which we soar; To the nursing faculty, without whom any of this would be possible; To our colleagues and the administrators at our respective universities who have helped pave the way, moved mountains, and given full support to integrating simulation within the nursing curriculum; To the nursing students at all levels: Excellence in nursing is not just a goal; it is a journey. Simulation can help take you there.

Contents

Part I: Setting the Foundation for Simulation

Part II: Innovative Simulation Scenarios in Diverse Settings

Part III: The Simulation Journey Continues

Contributors

Heather Bader, BSN, RN
Clinical Faculty
Educational Assistant
Three Rivers Community College
Norwich, Connecticut

Linda Bolin, RN, MSN, ANP
Clinical Associate Professor
East Carolina University
College of Nursing
Greenville, North Carolina

Carolynn Bruno, MS, RN
Assistant Professor of Nursing
Western Connecticut State
   University
Department of Nursing
Danbury, Connecticut

Chad M. Carson, RN, BSN
Regional Vice President of Sales
Emergisoft Corporation
Chicago, Illinois

Tamara L. Congdon, RN, BSN
Nursing Education Instructor
East Carolina University
College of Nursing
Greenville, North Carolina

Julie DeValk, BSN, RN
Pediatric Staff Nurse
Yale-New Haven Children's
   Hospital
New Haven, Connecticut

**Laura T. Gantt, RN, PhD, CEN,
   CNA, BC**
Executive Director
Learning Technologies and Labs
East Carolina University
College of Nursing
Greenville, North Carolina

Robin Goodrich, MS, RNC
Assistant Professor of Nursing
Department of Nursing
Western Connecticut State University
Danbury, Connecticut

Philip A. Greiner, DNSc, RN
Associate Professor of Nursing
Associate Dean of Public Health and
   Entrepreneurial Initiatives
Fairfield University
Fairfield, Connecticut

**Sheila Grossman, PhD, FNP,
   APRN-BC**
Professor of Nursing
Fairfield University
School of Nursing
Fairfield, Connecticut

**Pamela R. Jeffries DNS, RN, FAAN,
   ANEF**
Associate Dean of Undergraduate
   Programs
Indiana University School of Nursing
Indianapolis, Indiana

Alison Kris, PhD, RN
Assistant Professor
Fairfield University
School of Nursing
Fairfield, Connecticut

Jean W. Lange, PhD, RN
Associate Professor
Fairfield University
School of Nursing
Fairfield, Connecticut

Doris Troth Lippman, EdD, APRN, FAAN
Professor of Fairfield University
Fairfield University VA Academy
  Director
Fairfield University
School of Nursing
Fairfield, Connecticut

Diana DeBartolomeo Mager, MS, CRN
Director, Learning Resource Center
Fairfield University
School of Nursing
Fairfield, Connecticut

Laurence Miners, PhD
Professor of Economics
Director of Center for Academic
  Excellence
Fairfield University
Fairfield, Connecticut

Patricia Moreland, RN, CPNP, DNSc Candidate
Assistant Professor of Nursing
Department of Nursing
Western Connecticut State University
Danbury, Connecticut

Nancy A. Moriber, CRNA, MS, APRN
Program Director
Fairfield University and Bridgeport
  Hospital Nursing Anesthesia
  Program
Fairfield University
School of Nursing
Fairfield, Connecticut

Eileen R. O'Shea, DNP, RN
Assistant Professor
Fairfield University
School of Nursing
Fairfield, Connecticut

Michael P. Pagano, PA-C, PhD
Assistant Professor of Health
  Communications
Fairfield University
Fairfield, Connecticut

Lilian Rafeldt, RN, MA
Associate Professor of Nursing
Three Rivers Community
  College
Norwich, Connecticut

Catherine Rice, RN, EdD, CNA, BC
Associate Professor of Nursing
Western Connecticut State University
Department of Nursing
Danbury, Connecticut

Walter C. Robey III, MD
Director, Medical Simulation and
  Patient Safety Lab
Clinical Associate Professor
Department of Emergency
  Medicine
Brody School of Medicine
East Carolina University
Greenville, North Carolina

Joyce M. Shea, DNSc, APRN-BC, PMHCNS-BC
Assistant Professor of Nursing
School of Nursing
Fairfield University
Fairfield, Connecticut

Suzanne Turner, BSN, RN
Clinical Faculty
Educational Assistant
Three Rivers Community
  College
Norwich, Connecticut

Robin Webb Corbett, RN, C, PhD
Associate Professor
Capstone Course Coordinator
East Carolina University
College of Nursing
Greenville, North Carolina

Foreword

Timing is everything! With the explosion of the use and incorporation of simulations in nursing education today, this book, *Simulation Scenarios for Nurse Educators: Making It REAL!* could not have come at a better time. The 26-chapter book provides step-by-step guidelines for nursing faculty to design, develop, and implement clinical simulation scenarios in diverse settings, with diverse patients, and for different levels of students from the novice in a fundamentals course to the senior level critical care or capstone course.

The passion, caring, and inspiration of the authors is felt and delivered in each and every chapter. The book is based on the authors' personal experiences regionally and nationally with nursing faculty who have also experienced the frustrations, growing pains, and lack of knowledge about where to start when planning to incorporate simulations into a nursing course or curriculum. Compiling all of the authors' lessons learned, teaching-learning strategies, and in-depth research and exploration of their topics, this book is an excellent guide for nursing faculty just getting started with simulations or is validation for faculty who are already using this pedagogy.

Once you begin to read the book, you will not be able to put it down. As a first step in writing this foreword, I thought I would briefly scan through the chapters to have a view of the overall book and its components. However, I found the brief scan turned in to reading every page word for word. Many times, I nodded my head in agreement and smiled as I read material to which I could strongly relate.

Some of the highlights of the book are the beginning chapters by the co-editors on simulation pedagogy, integrating a simulation-focused pedagogy into the nursing curriculum, faculty learning communities, and how to integrate simulations into diverse settings. Various authors then provide chapters focusing on knowledge, strategies, and recommendations on how to implement simulations in different types of course or clinical settings. For example, if you are in doubt about how simulations can be incorporated in a physical assessment course, one chapter provides ideas, scenario objectives, and examples of how the simulation pedagogy can be used in this type of setting. The entire spectrum of courses from fundamentals, health assessment, and medical-surgical nursing courses, to more complex levels such as trauma resuscitation are discussed, with authors providing specific examples, simulation scenarios that include patient information, simulation objectives, preparation lists, and other information on all necessary components to develop and implement the simulation successfully. Various chapters address the diverse patient population including geriatric, pediatric, trauma, obstetric, and diabetic patients in terms of simulations that can be designed and implemented in those contexts. Finally, the last chapter of the book presents a cutting edge vision of the future of simulations which is appropriate since this teaching-learning pedagogy is changing almost on a daily basis affecting our nursing education and ultimately student learning and outcomes.

Timing is everything. As nursing leaders call for education reform to manage the shortage of clinical learning experiences, the lack of clinical sites, shortage of nurse educators, and the need to better prepare students for clinical decision making in a complex health care environment, this book provides practical solutions to begin the transformation of clinical education. The creativity and innovation demonstrated by the authors in this book on simulations provide a wonderful start to meeting these challenges. *Making it real* today is an important first step in contributing to tomorrow's future.

Pamela R. Jeffries, DNS, RN, FAAN, ANEF
Associate Dean of Undergraduate Programs
Indiana University School of Nursing

Preface

Nursing education is situated in a unique moment in time. In what has been called the *perfect storm* (Hinshaw, 2008), a faculty shortage has collided with a nursing shortage, and the two have resulted in challenges for nursing educators. Additionally, new generations of techno-savvy nursing students are before us in our classrooms. In the face of this challenge, nursing educators have the opportunity to create a new paradigm for teaching that reflects student need for interactive technology. Nurses have always responded to crises throughout time with creativity and innovation, and the same is true today. By complementing our traditional teaching with simulation, we, as educators, are addressing our need to do more with less. In making simulation *real*, we can deliver our teaching in an engaging yet effective manner, thereby transforming nursing education through a simulation-based pedagogy.

This book is divided into three parts. Part I provides an overview of the integration of simulation into nursing curricula, options for building a learning resource center, the description of innovative methods for faculty development related to integrating technology into the curriculum, and the role of health communication. Part II presents a collection of 17 exemplars containing actual scenarios in multiple clinical areas and testimonies of practicing faculty in a variety of settings at different levels of nursing education. It is meant to encourage nursing faculty that simulation development and incorporation into the curriculum is feasible and fun. The book provides concrete information about the use of simulation in a variety of programs, courses, and schools with flexible simulator uses, including live actors, static, and low-, medium-, and high-fidelity manikins. The practical applications are for those who are interested in taking first steps toward incorporating simulation or for those who have begun but want to expand beyond a typical medical-surgical, intensive care, and trauma focus. This book will encourage the development of critical thinking, clinical reasoning, and clinical judgment as well as caring, competent, safe practitioners. Finally, hints for suspending reality and "making it *real*" for students and faculty are incorporated throughout the book.

Finally, Part III explores future directions for simulations in nursing education. Given the work of the co-editors with the chapter authors and faculty in their own institutions, a framework of simulation learning was created and is provided in the final chapter of the book.

A template for creating scenarios is provided throughout the book, including the following:

- Student preparation materials, such as suggested readings, skills necessary for scenario enactment, and Web sites with more information

■ Forms to enhance the realness of the scenario, such as patient data forms, patient medication forms, and assessment tools (or Web sites where they can be acquired)

■ Checklists, such as health communication checklists to use in the creation of scenarios, evaluation criteria checklists for assessing student performance in scenarios, and debriefing guidelines.

The intent is to provide faculty with a strong basis to run multiple scenarios in a variety of clinical specialties geared at different learning levels and with different learning objectives. The supplemental materials provide easy access to materials for faculty and student use.

This long-awaited book provides *real* life stories of faculty in the trenches providing the light at the end of the tunnel to the sometimes challenging, but worthwhile, journey of simulation integration!

Reference

Hinshaw, A. S. (2008). Navigating the perfect storm: Balancing a culture of safety with workforce challenges. *Nursing Research, 57*(1S), S4–S10.

Acknowledgments

To all those who contributed time and effort in creating their scenarios for this book, we thank you from the bottom of our hearts for sharing your knowledge and expertise in describing your challenges and victories using simulation. There are numerous individuals who provided support. In grateful recognition, to name a few at Fairfield University: the administration, especially Dean Jeanne Novotny whose vision for the school has been an inspiration; Lab Director Diana Mager whose expertise in organizing, running, and overseeing the lab make this all possible, and colleague and co-director Phil Greiner, whose insight in so many areas has led to this greater vision; the School of Nursing Advisory Board, without whom this project would not have come to fruition, especially the chair Nancy Lynch, whose guidance and tireless perseverance has led to marvelous outcomes, and major donor Robin Kanarek, whose passion for nursing provides endless encouragement; Media Department Manager Kirk Anderson, who is always just a phone call away; the Center for Academic Excellence, especially Larry Miners, whose support for faculty development has been key to our progress, and the Computing and Network Services departments, as well as the students who have patiently worked with us throughout the years.

At Western Connecticut State University, grateful thanks are extended to Lorraine Capobianco and Kevin Koshel, whose work within University Computing have set the foundation for simulation; President James Schmotter, Provost Linda Rinker, and Dean Lynne Clark whose leadership and support have lead the way; Barbara Piscopo, who encouraged and supported the pursuit of simulation; Karen Crouse, who creatively and enthusiastically has embraced simulation in nursing education; Undergraduate Coordinator Deb Lajoie, as well as Kathy Barber and the Learning Resources Committee, who truly do all the work supporting simulation, and to the WCSU class of 2008 who inspired and created the student generated senior scenarios.

We cannot possibly name them all.

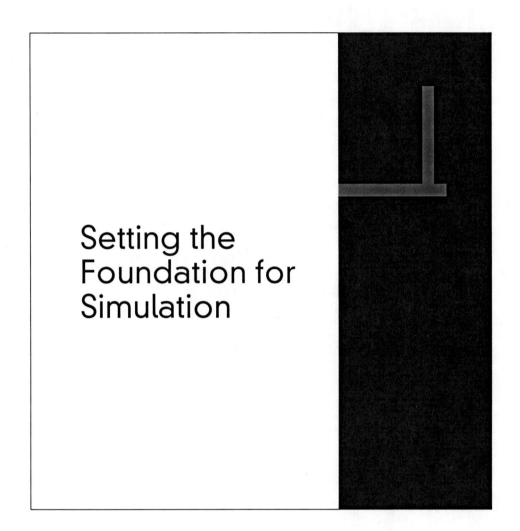

Setting the
Foundation for
Simulation

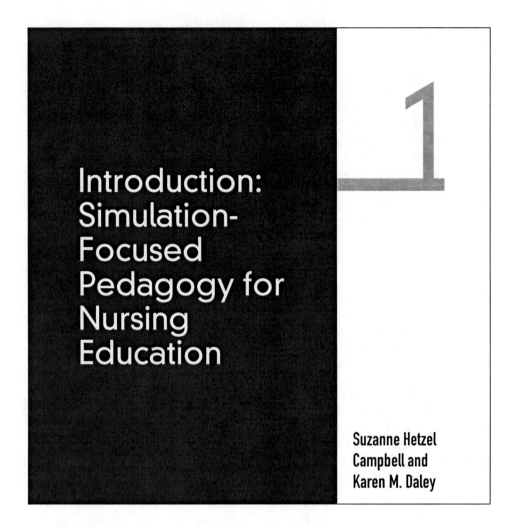

Introduction: Simulation-Focused Pedagogy for Nursing Education

1

Suzanne Hetzel
Campbell and
Karen M. Daley

Introduction

The Challenge of Teaching in the 21st Century

This book has been written related to our personal experiences regionally and nationally with audiences of nursing faculty who have expressed frustration, consternation, anxiety, and bewilderment about "where to start" with simulation, especially with human patient simulators. We have been privileged to be here at the start of simulation, with the inherent frustration of explaining to administration and fellow faculty the potential and vision that this innovative learning experience can provide for nursing students.

It is the hope of the editors that the simulations included in this text will provide nurse educators with a place to start—a template for the creation of their own broad and relevant experiences in the classroom and clinical settings. It is paramount that we share our passion for the process and our strong belief that all faculty can contribute, at whatever level of simulation, to this process. Yes, there are gaps in the literature and challenges expressed in the literature; yes, faculty struggles to meet the new demands of this technology within the realm of faculty shortages and workload. Yet the potential benefits to faculty and students are clear, especially by enhancing critical thinking beyond protocol and critical pathways. Oftentimes, it is an astute, expert nurse who, in noting subtle changes in his or her patient, enacts the kind of care that saves the patient's life. Nurses are the frontline providers of care.

Simulation enters here by allowing for reflection on all aspects of care. The built-in debriefing period, which encourages reflection on thoughts, actions, and outcomes, also leads to better transfer of content to practice and more versatile thinking processes for future application. In addition, the faculty role of mentor and facilitator in this process combines faculty expertise with student innovation. It is a learning process for all, which overall improves methods of teaching and learning.

Role of Simulation in Nursing Education

Nurse educators and researchers now recognize simulation as a valuable general tool for gaining knowledge (Alinier, Hunt, & Gordon, 2003; Childs & Sepples, 2006; Henneman & Cunningham, 2005; Jeffries, 2007; Roberts & McGowan, 2004). The availability of high-fidelity technology at reasonable cost, and the availability of funds to purchase this equipment, has resulted in widespread acquisition across the country. Some faculty, though, have reported to us that on delivery, these human patient simulators may remain in a box, unused. Other faculty, who have had the benefit of preassembly and attending 1- to 2-day workshops, need encouragement and inspiration to fully implement simulation within their individual courses. When attending simulation conferences, it appears that everyone is incorporating and using simulation (or has bought the equipment). But when you talk to faculty, they are confused, overwhelmed, and frustrated with trying to write and implement scenarios into their individual courses.

One only needs to watch a group of students in a simulation to fully appreciate the teaching and learning potentialities at hand. After all, simulation prompts positive results. However, the research for assessment and evaluation for nursing education falls behind the medical literature, and has not been fully tested and incorporated. For example, in a study of the use of clinical laboratories in Victoria, Australia (with site visits, interviews, and curricula review), researchers found that use of the laboratories was based on past experience, tradition, and resources rather than evidence (Wellard, Woolf, & Gleeson, 2007). Otherwise, while research on simulation in nursing is ongoing, it is still in its initial stages, just beyond description, and is still in need of synthesis. Of course, the benefits of simulation have been well documented by the National League for Nursing (NLN)/Laerdal simulation study (Jeffries & Rizzolo, 2005), and large projects have examined the benefits and best practice for implementation. But there is much more to learn.

On a broader level, administration finding the money for providing the necessary resources (faculty development, equipment purchase, building renovations, faculty time, etc.) does not transfer immediately into less faculty workload. In contrast, it often requires more investment of time and resources up front to get to the "work smarter, not harder" phase. One strategy has been to assign already overburdened lab directors with the "task" of incorporating simulation for faculty. Whether in static modules as testing prior to entering clinical, skill-based task training or end-point competency testing, the actual development and running of the scenarios is parceled out to lab staff, information technology personnel, and others. As this process may not directly involve faculty, their valuable educational and clinical expertise is more often overlooked. Another strategy allows for individual faculty to initiate simulation within their own teaching load in single courses. Faculty find this process time-consuming and complex when starting without help or guidance of those more experienced in simulation (Nehring & Lashley, 2004). Currently, experts in simulation are few and far between.

We feel that simulation offers an innovative approach that complements and easily integrates into existing nursing curricula, addressing the needs of a new generation of nurses and a society with increasingly complex health care needs. In order to fully appreciate the incorporation of simulation and the driving forces behind this movement, one needs to recognize that challenges include understanding issues facing nursing education, the influence of technology on theoretical and conceptual aspects of nursing education, learning in the digital culture, and the challenge of suspending belief to make simulations real. In order for a transfer of knowledge to occur, the student's role in the simulation needs to be as authentic as possible.

Some of the issues facing nursing education include the increased acuity level of patients, the nursing faculty and staff shortages, limited clinical sites, and the shifting role of the nurse. Quality and safety of patient care has become a major societal focus driving the increased accountability of nursing faculty and students to provide safe, effective, knowledgeable nurses who can function in a highly complex health care environment. Nurses are expected to demonstrate leadership skills in the coordination of patient care and safety and in this role oversee multidisciplinary teams who provide multifaceted care. Increasingly, nurses are expected to use their knowledge to transform health care delivery. Simulation provides an environment for the teaching and learning of multidisciplinary collaboration through scenarios embedded with communication, safety, delegation, critical thinking, and other important nursing program outcomes where novice nursing students can practice in a safe environment (Haskvitz & Koop, 2004; Jeffries, 2007; Radhakrishnan, Roche, & Cunningham, 2007). Finally, the challenge of assessment and evaluation of student performance can go beyond skill-based assessment and include processes such as student growth over time, development of critical thinking, and competencies of nursing education.

Theoretical and Conceptual Issues in Nursing Education

When viewed as a learning tool, simulation aligns well with the theoretical and conceptual foundations of nursing education. Models and frameworks have been proposed and utilized to help conceptualize the role of simulation in nursing education. One such model describes a simulation protocol that was formulated by the University of Maryland Baltimore School Of Nursing (Larew, Lessans, Spunt, Foster, & Covington, 2006). This protocol, based on the work of Benner (1984), utilizes a cue-based system with escalating prompts to move students through recognition to assessment to intervention to problem resolution.

Recommendations to highlight one problem at a time, allowing the scenarios to be student directed with time for processing in the pacing of the scenario, laid the foundation for further development of simulation frameworks. Jeffries and Rodgers (2007) propose a theoretical framework for simulation from "insights gained from theoretical and empirical literature" (p. 22) on simulation in nursing and related disciplines. This eclectic approach to formulating simulation frameworks provides the basis for a holistic, flexible, and multifaceted approach to integrating simulation into nursing education.

In addition to those seminal works cited above (Larew et al., 2006; Jeffries & Rodgers, 2007), we have considered the work of Tanner (2006) in our conceptualization of simulation. Tanner's model of clinical judgment is relevant in simulation because so much of what simulation is involves clinical judgment and decision making. Tanner's description of aspects of the process include noticing, interpreting, responding, and reflecting. This model emphasizes expectations of the situation that may be implicit or explicit. A particular emphasis on reflection finds support in the recent literature, which highlights reflection as an essential element in the improvement of clinical reasoning (Tanner). In simulation, an equivalent concept is debriefing, which should include Tanner's reflection-on-action as a synthesis of experiential knowledge resulting in formulation of best practices. In a clinical situation, nursing students often observe and are unable to enact interventions independently. In simulation, reflection on interventions can result in a second try in a safe environment, where improved outcomes are immediately evident.

Fink (2003), another driving force in our simulation-focused pedagogy, discusses the creation of significant learning experiences. Based in education research, he has compiled six major dimensions to "formulate significant learning goals" (Fink, p. 75). In considering these learning goals, we have identified areas that demonstrate how simulation complements nursing education to meet program goals and outcomes. For example, the goals include foundational knowledge (nursing content), application (enactment of the scenario allows for use of knowledge and skills in a safe environment), integration (synthesizing the science of nursing with knowledge from all disciplines—in conjunction with critical thinking, this dimension incorporates decision making and priority setting), human dimension (interacting with themselves and others to form a view of who they are as nursing professionals, including opportunities for collaboration), caring (the art of nursing), and learning how to learn (empowering students for professional lifelong learning). The debriefing component of simulation pedagogy allows for an integration of all six major dimensions of Fink's learning goals.

Of interest in simulation is social ecological theory (Stokols, 1996). This framework examines individual experiences and culture brought to social situations and how they impact behavioral outcomes. The social determinants of health (Wilkinson & Marmot, 2003), developed by the World Health Organization's European division in the 1990s, incorporates social ecological theory and was used as a foundation for Healthy People 2010 (U.S. Department of Health and Human Services, 2000). These theoretical cores should be directly linked to simulations as they are being developed.

For example, a common challenge for nurses working in inpatient environments is the decontextualization of the patient. By this, we mean that care is being provided without an understanding of the social and physical environment or the behavioral motivators related to health of the individual patient. The result can be that patient teaching and other nursing activities done in the institution do not match the reality of the patient's home environment. In home health care, nurses often need to reteach the patient and/or caregiver to fit the care plan to the resources available.

In simulation, not only is the context of the patient important, but educators must consider the cultural predispositions that students bring into the learning environment, which may affect behavior and the outcome of the scenario. Much the same is true within the culture of a nursing floor or unit. Clinical judgments made may be influenced by these multiple factors and need to be considered in culturally sensitive care of real patients. Also, simulations can be manipulated such that the patients being cared for have a variety of cultural backgrounds, needs, experiences, and diverse social and environmental support systems. Including these factors enhances the simulation and learning experience for students and increases the "realness" of the scenario.

Related nursing concepts in simulation are vigilance and failure to rescue. As nursing educators, vigilance is one of the most important yet difficult concepts to teach to nursing students (Almerud, Alapack, Fridlund, & Ekebergh, 2007; Jacobs, Apatov, & Glei, 2007; Meyer & Lavin, 2005). Although introduced early in assessment courses, the evolution of vigilance as an essential function of a nurse is amenable to practice and refinement during simulation. Once taught in this setting, students become aware of the value of maintaining vigilance in actual health care settings. A consequence of failed vigilance is failure to rescue. Although unethical to practice in the clinical setting, a student who experiences failure to rescue in a simulation can follow through with reflective debriefing, reformulate a plan, carry out the new plan, and then successfully maintain vigilance. Students have reported "never forgetting" the opportunity to "redo." Once again, this experience adds to the development of the student's vision of the impact of maintaining excellence in nursing care.

From the student perspective, there have been reports that conceptualizing the scenario through the lens of the nursing process while in the midst of a simulation is extremely helpful in producing positive outcomes! It has been frequently observed in our teaching that students, in the excitement of enacting a scenario, jump past focused assessments and begin performing interventions without data to support their decisions. Gentle coaching and reminders by the instructors alleviates this tendency.

In theorizing about technology in simulation, one may want to consider that beyond technological fidelity, there are actually three levels of fidelity: environmental, equipment and psychological (Fritz, Gray, & Flanagan, 2007).

- ■ *Environmental fidelity:* "The realism of the environment in which the simulation takes place" (Fritz et al., p. 2)
- ■ Equipment *fidelity:* "Hardware and/or software realism of the simulator" (Fritz et al., p. 2)
- ■ *Psychological fidelity:* "Reflects the degree to which the trainee perceives the simulation to be a believable representation of the reality it is duplicating" (Fritz et al., p. 2).

In nursing, we have incorporated these fidelities by making simulation as real as possible—a suspension of belief—so that the student interacts and participates more fully. The way space is structured to look and feel like a clinical unit, with necessary equipment, sets the scene for the simulation. In addition, events need to flow smoothly (e.g., responses from "patients" and "families") so that the student acknowledges his or her role in meeting patient needs.

There are three goals or levels of enacting a "reality-based" simulation:

1. *For students:* The simulation must be believable. They must take on the role of the "nurse" and feel the responsibility for the care, assessment, and delegation necessary to meet the needs of this "real" patient. If the patient takes a turn for the worse, can students believe that their actions (or inactions) may lead to an adverse outcome for the patient (maybe even death)? In reality, we would not want them to have a life-threatening experience with a real patient in clinical; however, simulation provides the safe environment to learn skills necessary for the prevention of adverse outcomes. It is necessary to "suspend reality" and allow the students to embrace their role and act confidently with the necessary critical reasoning to accomplish their objectives. The debriefing component of the simulation will be much richer if the students self-reflect from a perspective that their actions and decisions really made a difference in the outcome of care.

2. *For faculty:* Simulation must also be believable for faculty in the sense that they can accomplish this and meet their educational goals via simulation; it is feasible, possible, and fun. From learning theory and brain theory, we are trying to encourage the use of the right and left brain, which has been demonstrated to better embed the experience, and make the substance of what is learned more accessible or easily retrieved for use in future, varied, patient encounters (Seigel, 2007).

3. *Translation into practice:* Tapping into an emotional or psychological component for the students when learning has been demonstrated to improve memory and allow for better retrieving. Knowledge stored is better accessible and easily tapped for use in practice in a variety of situations. Students use a synthesis of past experiences to pool best practices into actual practice.

Learning in the Digital Culture

Technology in nursing education is here to stay. Today's students learn and study in the digital culture into which they were born. Multitasking is not an issue and, in fact, seems to be the way student brains are wired. Teaching to this group, whose attention span may be less than 10 to 15 minutes, requires new and innovative approaches other than the didactic. Repetitions, visual, and auditory and kinesthetic stimulation in an environment where students can move and interact while learning provide the variety of stimuli needed.

Of course, simulation also is one method to supplement didactic teaching. As such, educator expertise is essential when incorporating simulation. It requires background knowledge of the curriculum and the ability to assess where students should be, what they are capable of, and how nursing graduates from the program will function in the workforce. To provide optimal student learning experiences, changes in educational practices need to be incorporated with pedagogical principles, which in turn guide the development and implementation of simulation activities and the integration of technology (Jeffries, 2005). Simulation provides another avenue for achieving these outcome objectives. The importance of the integration of, exposure to, and mastery of technology has recently been confirmed and included in the revision of the *Essentials of Baccalaureate Education for Professional Nursing Practice* (American Association of Colleges of Nursing, 2007). For its part, the NLN (2003) challenges nursing to "reconceptualize reform in nursing education" by encouraging innovative teaching practices (p. 3).

Simulated patients allow for standardized learning experiences. Scenarios designed by nursing educators provide for focused learning with prescribed outcomes. Student performance can be measured and documented across groups and specific points of time in important focus areas of the curriculum. Results of these measurements can be used for assessment and evaluation progress toward curricular goals and program outcomes.

Murray, Grant, Howarth, and Leigh (2008) discuss the use of simulation for teaching and learning to support practice learning and state "simulation is a strategy to enhance clinical competence" (pp. 5–6). Used as a supplement to clinical preparation or for clinical remediation, simulation provides opportunities for students to practice clinical skills and interactions outside the actual patient setting. Kuiper, Heinrich, Matthias, Graham, and Kotwall (2008) concur, stating that the results of their study show that evidence "supports the use of simulation as a source of remediation for students with clinical challenges and for an enhancement of didactic content" (p. 12). Simulation has also been shown to increase the confidence of students in a low-anxiety setting prior to clinical experiences (Murray et al).

Simulation contributes to the development of the reflective practitioner who demonstrates better decision-making skills and superior problem-solving skills by using more creative thinking (Murray et al., 2008; Rauen, 2004). Unique to simulation exercises is the debriefing period, which allows for reflection on the effectiveness of interventions and processing of alternate theories for improving outcomes. Debriefing allows for reintegration of theory, evaluation of best practice, and an opportunity to learn about error management.

We are situated in a unique time period where the ability to use simulation fits with the issues of growing nursing faculty shortages and limited resources for student admission to programs as well as those related to clinical or agency use. In addition, safety and quality-of-care issues increase the importance of student education in situations where they can feel safe in providing care and transform an observational experience into a hands-on simulated learning experience.

As aptly put by Starkweather and Kardong-Edgren (2008), "the best outcomes with simulation occur when it is integrated across a curriculum, creating a challenge for academic nursing administrators, curriculum committees and faculty members who are struggling with how to incorporate simulation into, rather than on top of, already crowded curricular agendas" (p. 2). However, one must start at the beginning and often—simulation begins with one faculty in one course. This book explores the integration of simulation within a curriculum, building a learning resource center, an innovative approach to faculty development, and the role of health communication within simulation. In order to meet the needs of nurse educators who are looking for help with designing and implementing simulation, we have written and collected scenarios currently in use from several seasoned faculty. It is our hope that these exemplars will fuel and encourage those who are enthusiastic about integrating simulation within their nursing programs. Finally, Part III of this book explores future directions for simulations in nursing education and outlines a framework of simulation learning created by the co-editors of this book.

Conclusion

The "perfect storm" is near, and the survival of the profession of nursing and the outcome of health care is at risk. We strongly and biasly believe that simulation-focused pedagogy holds many rewards, but working through the challenges and the need for extra resources to incorporate it awaits us. Infusing our passion for the process and our love of teaching and learning is the goal of this book. If we can help even one faculty member enhance teaching to incorporate these ideas for interactive learning that engages and excites students, then our mission is complete.

References

Alinier, G., Hunt, W., & Gordon, R. (2003). Determining value of simulation in nurse education: Study design and initial results. *Nurse Education in Practice 4,* 200–207.

Almerud, S., Alapack, R. J., Fridlund, B., & Ekebergh, M. (2007). Of vigilance and invisibility— being a patient in a technologically intense environment. *Nursing in Critical Care, 12*(3), 151–158.

Association of Colleges of Nursing. (2007). The October 22, 2007 draft of the *essentials of baccalaureate education for professional nursing practice.* Washington, DC: AACN.

Benner, P. (1984). *From novice to expert: Excellence and power in clinical nursing practice.* Menlo Park, CA: Addison Wesley.

Childs, J. C., & Sepples, S. B. (2006). Lessons learned from a complex patient care scenario. *Nursing Education Perspectives, 27*(3), 154–158.

Fink, L. D. (2003). *Creating significant learning experiences: An integrated approach to designing college courses.* San Francisco, CA: Jossey-Bass.

Fritz, P. Z., Gray, T., & Flanagan, B. (2007). Review of mannequin-based high-fidelity simulation in emergency medicine. *Emergency Medicine Australasia, 20*(1), 1–9.

Haskvitz, L. M., & Koop, E. C. (2004). Students struggling in clinical? A new role for the human patient simulator. *Journal of Nursing Education, 43*(4), 181–184.

Henneman, E. A., & Cunningham, H. (2005). Using clinical to teach patient safety in an acute/critical care nursing course. *Nurse Educator, 30*(4), 172–177.

Jacobs, J. L., Apatov, N., & Glei, M. (2007). Increasing vigilance on the medical/surgical floor to improve patient safety. *Journal of Advanced Nursing, 57*(5), 472–481.

Jeffries, P. (2007). *Simulation in nursing education.* New York: National League for Nurses.

Jeffries, P. R. (2005). A framework for designing, implementing and evaluating simulations used as teaching strategies in nursing. *Nursing Education Perspectives, 26*(2), 96–103.

Jeffries, P. R., & Rizollo, M. A. (2006). Designing and implementing models for the innovative use of simulation to teach nursing care of ill adults and children: A national, multi-site, multi-method study. In P. Jeffries (Ed.), *Simulation in nursing education* (pp. 145–159). New York: National League for Nurses.

Jeffries, P. R., & Rodgers, K. J. (2007). Theoretical framework for simulation design. In P. Jeffries (Ed.), *Simulation in nursing education* (pp. 21–33). New York: National League for Nurses.

Kuiper, R. A., Heinrich, C., Matthias, A., Graham, M. J., & Kotwall, L. B. (2008). Debriefing with the OPT model of clinical reasoning during high-fidelity patient simulation. *International Journal of Nursing Education Scholarship, 17*(5), 1–14.

Larew, C., Lessans, S., Spunt, D., Foster, D., & Covington, B. G. (2006). Application of Benner's theory in an interactive simulation. *Nursing Education Perspectives, 27*(1), 16–21.

Meyer, G., & Lavin, M. A. (2005). Vigilance: The essence of nursing. *Online Journal of Issues in Nursing, 10*(3), 38–51.

Murray, C., Grant, M. J., Howarth, M. L., & Leigh, J. (2008). The use of simulation as a teaching and learning approach to support practice learning. *Nurse Education in Practice, 8*(1), 5–8.

National League for Nursing. (2003). *Position statement. Innovation in nursing education: A call to reform.* Retrieved April 26, 2008, from http://www.nln.org/aboutnln/PositionStatements/innovation.htm

Nehring, W. M., & Lashley, F. R. (2004). Human patient simulations in nursing education: An international survey. *Nurse Education in Practice, 25*(5), 244–248.

Radhakrishnan, K., Roche, J. P., & Cunningham, H. (2007). Measuring clinical practice parameters with human patient simulators: A pilot study. *International Journal of Nursing Education Scholarship, 4*(1), 1–10.

Rauen, C. A. (2004). Cardiovascular surgery: Simulation as a teaching strategy for nursing education and orientation in cardiac surgery. *Critical Care Nurse, 24*(3), 46–51.

Roberts, S. W., & McGowan, R. J. (2004). The effectiveness of infant simulations. *Adolescence, 39*(155), 475–487.

Seigel, D. (2007). *The mindful brain: Reflection and attunement in the cultivation of well-being.* New York: WW Norton & Company.

Starkweather, A. R., & Kardong-Edgren, S. (2008). Diffusion of innovation: Embedding simulation into nursing curricula. *International Journal of Nursing Education Scholarship, 5*(1), 1–11.

Stokols, D. (1996). Translating social ecological theory into guidelines for community health promotion. *American Journal of Health Promotion, 10,* 282–298.

Tanner, C. (2006). Thinking like a nurse: A research based model of clinical judgment in nursing. *Journal of Nursing Education, 45*(6), 204–211.

Wellard, S. J., Woolf, R., & Gleeson, L. (2007). Exploring the use of clinical laboratories in undergraduate nursing programs in regional Australia. *International Journal of Nursing Education Scholarship, 4*(1). Retrieved February 13, 2008, from http://www.bepress.com/ijnes/vol4/iss1/art4

Wilkinson, R., & Marmot, M. (2003). *Social determinants of health: The solid facts* (2nd ed.). Copenhagen, Denmark: World Health Organization.

U.S. Department of Health and Human Services. (2000). With understanding and improving health and objectives for improving health. *Healthy people 2010* (2nd ed.). Washington, DC: U.S. Government Printing Office.

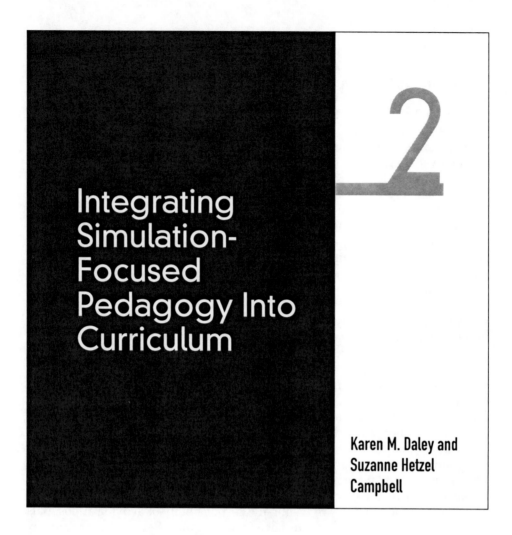

Integrating Simulation-Focused Pedagogy Into Curriculum

2

Karen M. Daley and
Suzanne Hetzel
Campbell

This chapter will describe how simulation fits the needs for 21st-century nursing education. Aspects to be covered include the changing needs for nursing education in a technologically complex environment, how to succeed when incorporating simulation, the importance of the faculty role in embedding simulation throughout the nursing curriculum, meeting the challenges of clinical placement, and specific challenges and benefits to integrating simulation into the curriculum with an evidence-based practice focus.

Simulation: The Missing Piece

Historically, education at all levels has emphasized critical thinking as a standard. Students now arrive on campus with the basic skills to learn through critical thinking. However, distinct to this generation of learners is the ability to use and adapt readily to the rapid technological advances seen since the turn of the century. Although primarily used as a source of entertainment and creativity, these students often arrive knowing more about technology than their teachers and expecting nontraditional teaching methods that incorporate technology at every turn. As always, the challenge on the college campuses for faculty is to stay abreast, if not ahead of, a typical undergraduate's technology-laden learning needs in addition to facilitating the higher level of critical thinking expected of college graduates. Simulation provides the missing piece for nursing education through harnessing each student's enthusiasm for technology into an interactive and valuable learning experience in which to engage in critical thinking (Radhakrishnan, Roche, & Cunningham, 2007).

The last 10 years have seen major advancements in technology available in nursing education, and most faculty and nursing programs have recognized the need for incorporating technology into the way they are teaching. Teachers now have technology-equipped classrooms that have the capability to use streamlined video, have in-classroom Web access, and use Web-based learning platforms in each class, and students are encouraged to "Google." Virtual hospitals have appeared online, interactive nursing case studies are readily available, and we now have the ability to stream actual patient data in real time into remote classrooms for analysis. In addition, in the last 10 years, high-technology products have become available for students to learn nursing in lifelike patient encounters. Most recently, with the creation of high-fidelity human patient simulators, there is an opportunity to take simulation to a higher interactive level within the bounds of practice and safety prior to actual patient interactions. This technology is within reach of most nursing programs from the traditionally basic level to the most cutting edge.

However, navigating the simulation maze, obtaining and renovating space, and, most importantly, obtaining faculty buy-in and promoting ownership of simulation within the curriculum have not proved to be a smooth transition. Presently, the need for more complicated scenarios has evolved as patients have become sicker and staff nurses have been required to provide more complex care. Nursing faculty who are feeling the responsibility of arriving at hospitals with competently trained students have identified the need to practice complex care prior to clinical experiences. Simulation meets this need.

The traditional approach to the use of simulation in nursing curricula is to develop independent modules that students must complete and be "assessed" on prior to entering the clinical areas. Traditionally, low-fidelity simulations on static manikins has been delivered by lab personnel under the direction of faculty. These scenarios are easily set up, require low maintenance materials, and allow for easy evaluation. These methods have a long history of proven success in task training and may or may not involve individual nursing faculty input. However, task-based modules such as catheterization do not require the same level of complexity, critical thinking, communication, and use of nursing skills as a scenario that integrates all these areas.

In contrast, the simulations provided in this book come from competent clinical and seasoned faculty who have been actively integrating simulation into every course taught. This feature brings a new level of curricular sophistication and provides an example for others of how methods they are using to teach already can be incorporated with a simulation-focused pedagogy. Throughout the text, the term *simulation-focused pedagogy* is used to describe a method of utilizing simulation and scenarios to integrate content and multiple concepts in all areas of nursing care to provide an interactive environment by which students are held accountable to use the information they are learning. Simulation integrates theoretical didactic components with critical thinking to enact nursing behaviors in a safe, efficient, ethical manner or as an end point (capstone) measure of competencies. Although simulation-focused pedagogy has become a worthy and essential curricular goal, most nursing educators have struggled to find ways to integrate simulation throughout each program's curriculum.

Other literature has emphasized purely medical and surgical uses for simulation; however, we feel strongly that simulation crosses all clinical areas of nursing curricula and is applicable in all areas. All faculty are capable of being involved in the development, implementation, and evaluation of scenarios to meet their curricular goals. The scenarios presented provide a wide breadth of simulation scenarios for all levels of undergraduate nursing curricula.

The Essential Tool Kit for Success: Persistence, Vision, and Patience

Many of us have arrived at simulation in one of two ways: as a dream for how things should be done with little or no financing or as a well-financed initiative with no schematics for implementation of something designated as the "simulation lab." However, as one arrives at simulation, the realization occurs quickly that this has been a daunting task to implement. Many levels arise for implementation, and hidden costs and factors are continually discovered. Yet, once implemented, the results are amazing.

Our joint experience is that persistence in pursuing the implementation of simulation is invaluable. One faculty member described this as a "dogged" and unrelenting pursuit! Whether the vision has been dictated or created individually, it is this vision that will help to climb the many walls and meet the pitfalls and challenges that arise head on. Patiently reiterating the need, returning to key people to explain the rationale and vision, and writing and rewriting plans and strategies have been required throughout the experience. Key to this persistence has been the support, encouragement, and faith of faculty.

The Faculty Factor

Building a foundation for the integration of simulation throughout the curriculum must take into account the faculty factor. Although most who are leading the way for integration of simulation are comfortable with the technology, most nursing faculty groups reflect varying levels of technology training and utilization of technology in their classes. High-fidelity simulation requires more than a basic understanding of computers. Most simulation companies who were initially willing to train faculty as needed are now charging for this service, necessitating a "train the trainers" type of initiative. This often forces a decision to find an expert or two who, in addition to a usual faculty load, will then be responsible for training the entire faculty on how to use the simulators—a very daunting task. Finding time for individual or group training is essential but can be difficult to manage given the faculty shortages and already busy workload of nursing faculty. Because not all nursing programs have lab personnel, often individual faculty must be trained to run their own simulations. However, promoting ownership and individual buy-in within a faculty member's program or course and group simulation initiatives often eases the transition to integrating simulation into individual courses. Given the atmosphere of academic freedom, some strategies to encourage and inspire hesitant faculty may include inviting them to observe a scenario or role-play one of the parts; having an "open door" policy for interested faculty to discuss their ideas, outline templates, and receive coaching in simulation; retreats to strategize about methods to embed simulation and technology throughout the curriculum; and faculty learning communities (see chapter 4).

Clinical Versus Simulation

The need for simulated nursing experiences has been reinforced by the scarcity of clinical placement sites. As programs have increased enrollment, the large numbers of students needing clinical experiences and a nursing shortage that requires adequate staffing to handle students have created stress for both academic institutions and hospitals alike. This situation has sparked much discussion about how much clinical time should be replaced with simulation or whether simulation should ever replace clinical time at all. Although most nursing programs are deciding this issue individually, each program has required hours for program completion by individual state boards of nursing. In one state, a brainstorming session of the statewide deans and directors was held early in this new era of simulation, and in general, it was suggested that no more than 10% of clinical time would be used for simulation. Other states have made arrangements for incorporating simulation into calculated clinical time. The National Council of State Boards of Nursing (NCSBN) Position paper of 2005 reported that boards addressed two major issues: the increased use of technology for nursing education clinical experiences and the use of clinical sites and learning centers. Although nursing education experiences should be across the life span with actual patients, they may include innovative teaching strategies that complement clinical, like simulation but should not entirely replace clinical. In reality, with practice time in the simulation lab, students may enter the clinical sites at a higher cognitive and skill level with increased confidence and therefore get more out of the experience (Bremner, Aduddell, Bennett, & VanGeest, 2006; Murray, Grant, Howarth, & Leigh, 2008; NCSBN, 2005; Nehring, 2008).

A frequently used method of integrating simulation as a complement to clinical is doing simulations early in the semester. Nursing faculty are often unfamiliar with a new group of students and need to assess their competency level prior to placing these students with actual patients. The use of simulated scenarios can help prepare students for the higher level of patient care required in a new semester. Faculty can then move forward into the semester having assessed strengths, weaknesses, and areas in need of improvement.

Another method of implementing simulation within a semester is transforming what currently exists in the form of weekly task-oriented modules to simulation scenarios. Traditionally used to demonstrate competency on one static task, simulations transform a static task into an engaging and realistic patient interaction involving communication, safety precautions, and the need to react to changing physiologic conditions. In addition, when hospitals have the available resources (e.g., high-fidelity patient simulators), clinical faculty may choose to incorporate a simulation into postconference to share an important learning experience with the whole group, reinforce important aspects of care, and debrief to assist the students in recognizing alternative scenarios for providing care and assessing and evaluating patient reaction to the plan of care and actual nursing interventions.

Simulation has also been used for clinical remediation when a student is struggling in clinical (Bremner et al., 2006; Haskvitz & Koop, 2004; Kuiper, Heinrich, Matthias, Graham, & Kotwall, 2008). A student can be assigned time in the lab with a simulator, to reprocess a difficult clinical situation, to practice a skill that she or he was unable to perform in clinical, and/or to re-create an actual patient situation that a student needs to process more slowly in order to understand. Providing an opportunity where students can process in a safe environment often increases a student's confidence in actual patient interactions. From an assessment standpoint, if a student is not safe and not meeting the objectives in clinical, simulation can help both the faculty and student pinpoint deficits in critical thinking and decision making.

Faculty have also found simulations to be useful as an end point assessment of knowledge learned. Simulation testing can be used at the close of the semester as a final competency assessment or as a program assessment prior to graduation (see chapter 20). Hospitals have now begun testing minimum competencies of both new graduates and new hires using simulators and scenarios. End point simulation testing has better prepared new graduates for this challenge.

Formal Curricular Change Versus Integration Into the Existing Curriculum

We have heard many faculty discuss the fact that adding simulation would require a major and formal change in their program curriculum. We respectfully disagree. Simulation is, simply, a learning tool. We have been using simulation since the practice of teaching nursing began. We used each other in nursing school to learn our assessments, practiced static skills on static manikins, and gave injections to oranges. Certainly, computerized simulation is at a different level, but we have found that other than adding or rewording some course objectives or retooling a practice module to a technology-enhanced module, there has not been a need to rewrite the curriculum. As time passes, we feel there may be a need on a graduate level to add a course on technology-based learning that may include simulation. However, most programs have been able to seamlessly add simulation as a within-course learning experience.

Establishing the Fit Across the Curriculum

The goal of simulation has been to enhance critical thinking and decision making at all levels of a nursing curriculum through realistic interactions with a simulated patient. Simulation can be implemented in every course, although some aspects of this implementation depend on the availability of faculty who are able to join in the scenario (possibly running the simulation equipment, being a disconcerted family member, or even being the voice of the patient). At a sophomore or program-entry level, uses for simulation include physical assessment within the first medical-surgical course and in studying pharmacology. In learning physical assessment, students can use simulation to assess body sounds, locate landmarks, and run and rerun system assessments as needed for enhancing learning. In a lower-level medical-surgical course, students can interact with the simulated patient prior to meeting patients and practice communication techniques. An instructor may decide to introduce a difficult patient scenario to a novice nursing student so that strategies for success can be practiced prior to meeting an actual challenging patient. Simulation has been used in teaching pharmacology to bring home the seriousness of prioritizing a patient's safety in medication administration (Seropian, Dillman, Lasater, & Givilanes, 2007). Using a high-fidelity human patient simulator, an instructor has the capacity to show real-time effects of a medication as it is administered. Within a scenario, the instructor can show the positive effects as well as the side effects of certain mediations while demonstrating the physiologic impact of that medication in specific disease categories.

In mid-level curriculum or at the junior level, simulation can be utilized in the application of the nursing process throughout the life span. Simulation scenarios can be developed in chronic and acute medical surgical care, family care, care of mother and baby, pediatrics, geriatrics, home care, and psychiatric care. These scenarios can be tailored to involve multiple students and faculty enacting various family and professional roles in order to demonstrate the complexity of holistic care.

At the senior level, simulation is effective in teaching the application of the nursing process in complex and emergency nursing care (Childs & Sepples, 2006; Comer, 2005). Although impractical and unethical to wait until an actual patient situation becomes an emergency, student responses to emergency and life-threatening simulated scenarios can be assessed through the use of simulation. These scenarios can be run or programmed to have multiple outcomes depending on the student actions within the scenario. While many dispute the ethics of letting a simulator flatline in a scenario, simulations that test a student's knowledge in resuscitation, either alone or in a team, have been reported to be important learning experiences for students who are able to practice their first code on a simulated patient. Although students verbalize disappointment when the outcome is not positive, they are very enthusiastic about running and rerunning the scenario until a positive outcome is achieved. This experience is unique to the high-fidelity simulators. In contrast, if a positive outcome is not achieved, students are provided the opportunity to practice good communication skills with family members and broach topics of organ donation, spirituality, and proper protocol for pronouncement of death and management of the body. Even though these are perceived as challenging situations to enact, graduates often identify such situations as areas in which they wish there had been more instruction while in nursing school so that they would be properly prepared for their real-life experiences as a nurse.

Although most scenarios are generated by faculty for use in their own courses, simulations have also been developed by students, as suggested by Larew, Lessans, Spunt, Foster, and Covington (2006). At all levels of the curriculum, students can be encouraged to use actual patient data to build their own scenario for their own learning as well as for demonstration purposes for the class (see chapter 22 for an example of student-generated senior scenarios). One university professor is using student-developed studies in the pediatric clinical rotation. As it is often challenging to find high-acuity pediatric patients on a consistent basis in any clinical setting, this professor instructs the students to generate a complex scenario as a replacement or supplement to actual patients cared for. Students then demonstrate for the class and submit a paper summary for grading. The person who specializes in simulation works with the students to familiarize them with the medium-fidelity manikin as part of the project, but learning the ins and outs of running the technology is part of the learning experience.

As another example, in a women's health course, students in groups are responsible for presenting specific case scenarios on key areas such as ectopic pregnancy and preterm labor. They are given some basic guidelines of information but are responsible for researching the clinical condition, identifying the nurse's role, and coming up with an appropriate care plan. This method can involve role-play or the use of simulated patients, and their peers are more engaged when involved in this style of interactive learning. From here, the faculty go on to incorporate content-appropriate material and reinforce the important points that all the students can relate back to with the benefit of a concrete "scenario."

Evidence-Based Practice

An essential component to integrating simulation throughout the curriculum is the inclusion of evidence-based practice throughout. Scenarios should include reference lists of research studies and standards of care used (Childs, Sepples, & Chambers, 2007). Prior to, during, and after simulations, students should also have access to resources for finding additional information needed to complete or understand the scenario. Just as is true in nursing care of real patients, students should be using only the latest research in the implementation of care on the simulated patient. Students may be asked in advance to pull standards of care and research prior to simulations. Students may have access to the Web through the classroom computer, a personal digital assistant, or a tablet computer. Also, many programs have set up simulation Web sites for use by the students and faculty in learning more about the simulation process and for quick access to important Web sites as references. For faculty, it is helpful if a scenario references the National Council Licensure Examination for a Registered Nurse (NCLEX-RN) categories (NCSBN, 2007) and/or accreditation bodies such as the American Association of Colleges of Nursing (AACN) and its *Essentials of Baccalaureate Education for Professional Nursing Practice* (AACN, 1998) and current revisions, for curricular reference points.

Benefits Across the Curriculum

The benefits of integrating simulation in selected courses throughout the curriculum are immediately evident: Students respond enthusiastically to the technology but more importantly are able to accurately diagnose and intervene in nursing problems beyond faculty expectations. Because of the breadth of programming of the medium- and high-fidelity simulation manikins, faculty no longer have to search for actual patients with all heart, lung, and abdominal problems and abnormal sounds. This allows for recognition of an assessment factor already learned prior to actual patient care, significantly increasing the likelihood of accurate assessment while caring for actual patients. In addition, students can be exposed to more conditions in a more controlled environment at a more rapid pace. Simulation takes on a life of its own, thus becoming "real" to the students.

References

American Association of Colleges of Nursing. (1998). *Essentials of baccalaureate education for professional nursing practice*. Retrieved February 2, 2008, from http://www.aacn.nche.edu/Education/pdf/BaccEssentials98.pdf

Bremner, M. N., Aduddell, K., Bennett, D. N., & VanGeest, J. B. (2006). The use of human patient simulators: Best practices with novice nursing students. *Nurse Educator, 31*(4), 170–174.

Childs, J. C., & Sepples, S. B. (2006). Lessons learned from a complex patient care scenario. *Nursing Education Perspectives, 27*(3), 154–158.

Childs, J. C., Sepples, S. B., & Chambers, K. (2007). Designing simulation for nursing education. In P. Jeffries (Ed.), *Simulation in nursing education* (pp. 35–58). New York: National League for Nurses.

Comer, S. (2005). Role playing to enhance clinical understanding. *Nursing Education Perspectives, 26*, 357–360.

Haskvitz, L. M., & Koop, E. C. (2004). Students struggling in clinical? A new role for the human patient simulator. *Journal of Nursing Education, 43*, 181–184.

Kuiper, R. A., Heinrich, C., Matthias, A., Graham, M. J., & Kotwall, L. B. (2008). Debriefing with the OPT model of clinical reasoning during high-fidelity patient simulation. *International Journal of Nursing Education Scholarship, 17*(5), 1–14.

Larew, C., Lessans, S., Spunt, D., Foster, D., & Covington, B. G. (2006). Application of Benner's theory in an interactive simulation. *Nursing Education Perspectives, 27*(1), 16–21.

Murray, C., Grant, M. J., Howarth, M. L., & Leigh, J. (2008). The use of simulation as a teaching and learning approach to support practice learning. *Nurse Education in Practice, 8*, 5–8.

National Council of State Boards of Nursing. (2005). *Clinical instruction in prelicensure nursing programs*. Retrieved May 2, 2008, from https://www.ncsbn.org/Final_Clinical_Instr_Pre_Nsg_programs.pdf

National Council of State Boards of Nursing. (2007). *NCLEX-RN Examination: Test Plan for the National Council Licensure Examination for Registered Nurses*. Retrieved June 18, 2008, from https://www.ncsbn.org/RN_Test_Plan_2007_Web.pdf

Nehring, W. M. (2008). U.S. boards of nursing and the use of high-fidelity patient simulators in nursing education. *Journal of Professional Nursing, 24*(2), 109–117.

Radhakrishnan, K., Roche, J. P., & Cunningham, H. (2007). Measuring clinical practice parameters with human patient simulators: A pilot study. *International Journal of Nursing Education Scholarship, 4*(1), 1–10.

Seropian, M., Dillman, D., Lasater, K., & Gavilanes, J. (2007). Mannequin-based simulation to reinforce pharmacology concepts. *Simulation in Healthcare, 2*(4), 218–223.

3

Building a Learning Resource Center

Karen M. Daley,
Suzanne Hetzel
Campbell, and Diana
DeBartolomeo
Mager

Traditionally, nursing programs have taught and practiced technical skills in a "nursing lab." As time has passed and technology has evolved, these labs have expanded to include computer stations, Web access, and computer-based learning platforms for skill acquisition. Today, nursing labs often contain all the resources needed for teaching and learning nursing skills through integrated processes that include mock-ups of a hospital. In addition, the technology in the nurse's practice setting is growing and expanding at an exponential rate. Computers are used for fully computerized charting and for interfacing with all departments and personnel. For many hospitals, test results and orders are delivered via computer. In addition, many nursing stations—once essential as a place for nursing documentation—have been replaced with individual computers on wheels, called *COWS,* for each nurse for each shift. Each semester and each clinical placement for the student presents faculty and students with technologic challenges that change every semester. New computerized equipment and care systems abound. It has become essential that any nursing lab, frequently called a *learning resource center,* includes the latest state-of-the-art equipment for patient care as well as patient care delivery systems. It is no longer adequate for students to just show up and perform basic nursing tasks but is essential for students to become an active part of the simulated learning environment in order to learn.

To that end, nursing programs are finding that the traditional lab is inadequate to meet the needs of today's students. Technology has become a necessary means to support, deliver, and evaluate nursing competencies. Skill-based education is still essential and can be delivered through static and computerized learning modules. However, preparation of students for a complex health care environment requires that students are educated not only in skills but also in communication, safety, and collaborative care. Varied levels of technology assist in this endeavor. Whether static, low fidelity, medium fidelity, or high fidelity, all should be available to assist students in meeting learning objectives.

Envisioning a Center

Many programs have worked diligently to expand, room by room, from a nursing lab to a learning resource center. These centers include simulation labs, static skill labs, resource libraries with nursing references, and ideally a computer lab. Several programs have benefited from large grants that allowed architectural design and construction of the ideal environment. In either case, creating a vision and a plan is essential. Other schools have creatively used available space to alter the methods with which they provide simulation education. However, no amount of planning guarantees a smooth transition from lab to center.

The needs of a program shift quickly with enrollment changes, which challenges simulation practice space and classroom use. As enrollment increases and expansion of program courses extend into summer and intersession time periods, lab spaces need to be easily accessible to meet the needs of a variety of courses. The flexibility of the space is of utmost importance. The objective of providing a multifaceted learning experience must be the foundation of any learning resource center endeavor.

The vision for the center should not be a one-person quest, although often that is exactly how the journey starts. Faculty buy-in is crucial! Otherwise the human patient simulators (HPS) may become nothing more than "very expensive paperweights" (Dean Jeanne Novotny, personal communication). Communicating the need campuswide is an additional challenge. As no man is an island, no department exists alone. Many departments will be involved in the successful implementation of a learning resource center.

When considering the needs of the faculty, students, and curriculum, envisioning the center requires outlining areas of importance. These areas include space issues, equipment needs, technology, support personnel (lab, information technology [IT], students), funding, and faculty development. One way of prioritizing these needs is to create a "wish list" to help identify what is realistic given situational factors.

When creating a wish list, consider dividing it into the following sections:

- *Grand wish list:* Things you would get if you had unlimited funds
- *Desired wish list:* Items that the faculty specifically request for courses

■ *Realistic wish list:* Prioritize the grand wish list and the desired wish list to match the actual funding and budget for purchase order development

Space issues, lab layouts and consideration of needs, and flexibility of space may include the following:

■ Furniture that is easily mobile (stackable, rolling)
■ Storage units for equipment and other resources
■ Computer technology to meet multiple needs, including a faculty console with DVD, CD, VCR, computer, and write-on board options; wireless capability; an LCD projector; and, if possible, taping, recording, and podcasting options
■ Interchangeable classrooms for lecture, computer-assisted instruction, small group interaction, health assessment, technical skill performance, group presentation, and simulation scenarios

Learning Resource Room or Center Essentials for Simulation Learning

No two nursing labs or learning resource centers are ever the same. When conceptualizing your center, important considerations include the following:

■ Available space (e.g., is it shared with other university programs?)
■ Large lab room versus multiple smaller rooms or areas
■ Determination of the number of specialty rooms or areas, such as medical-surgical, intensive care unit [ICU], operating room [OR], pediatrics, women's health, home care, long-term care
■ The relevance of lab needs to the present nursing curriculum (e.g., how many classes at a time will need the space, at what points in the semester, and during what time frames)
■ Incorporation of other components or threads, such as communication, palliative care, leadership, delegation, and documentation
■ Specific equipment needs
■ A vision that incorporates input from faculty, administration, and students—buy-in is crucial at all levels
■ Availability of lab personnel to assist with setting up and running the scenario
■ Use of volunteers to role-play (visual and performing arts students, members of the American Association of Retired Persons [AARP], retired doctors and nurses, health communication faculty or majors, other students and faculty)
■ Faculty resources for curriculum development and planning (Center for Academic Excellence, Scholarship of Teaching and Learning Centers)
■ Use of the School of Business to help with the development of a plan for sustainability
■ IT and media support

Early in the process of developing a center, one HPS may be used for multiple purposes, but over time, we have found it best to designate specialty areas in order to focus on specific learning experiences. Setting up simulation labs so that the specialty-specific simulation area is self-contained may be preferable (e.g., a pediatric area should have all pediatric equipment needed for scenarios and teaching). Should the rooms be separated by larger distances (e.g., separate buildings), one might find it necessary to duplicate equipment for both areas. Ideally, the simulation area should be a classroom-size area with a cart or cabinets that have room for all necessary equipment. If possible, having a classroom nearby with projection capability to record and project live-time scenario enactment from the simulation rooms would be the ideal. In this situation, the larger classroom could function as a learning environment to allow the knowledge transfer from simulation to the classroom and eventually from the classroom to hands-on care. In a separate venue, the participants in the simulation need time for debriefing of the scenario where a small group can sit to discuss specifics about its role and how things might go differently.

In addition, having a resource area is helpful, where copies of textbooks and references are available so that students can readily access the information needed to meet their learning goals during the simulation. Often, when students have an opportunity to "redo", this reference area facilitates the processing of an unsuccessful scenario. Students can search for solutions on site and use the computers available.

Props that enhance the "realness" of the scenario are helpful as well such as stretchers, charts, a crash cart, a defibrillator, an electrocardiogram (EKG) machine, intravenous (IV) solutions, lines and machines., The room or area should feel *real* as much as possible to enhance the authenticity of the scenario. Students should feel less like they are "playing pretend" and more like this simulation could really be happening. Of course, once the simulation starts, it often takes on a life of its own! In order to further enhance the realness, the setup needs to be efficient. The key to successful scenarios is to be able to set up quickly and dress the manikin for success with wounds, a Foley and IV, medications, a chart, and equipment nearby. One idea is to put together grab-and-go packets or plastic bins for each scenario so that assembly and take-down time are minimal. The packets or bins should be nearby in a cabinet or treatment-type cart for easy portability. Technical equipment such as video and sound equipment and various computers should not be noticeable. Many programs use control rooms with a one-way mirror or have the scenario controller behind a curtain. However, with the addition of the personal digital assistant remote access on some HPS, the person controlling the scenario can be nearby or in the scene making rapid click-and-go adjustments to the scenario as it progresses.

Considering the high expense of these medium- and high-fidelity HPS, having a plan for downtime usage becomes important as time passes. Often, HPS use is somewhat seasonal depending on course rotations, so making the most of using the HPS is key. Partnering with outside agencies for staff training, updating skills, accreditation standards, and/or new staff competency training allows collaboration with local key groups. Using the simulation lab as an income-generating entity during low usage times is always a possibility as well as donating use of the facility to agencies that have gone above and beyond accommodating student placements. Also, in the summer months, the simulation labs and learning resource center can be used for accelerated programs, graduate courses, and continuing education programs.

Karen's Story: Western Connecticut State University Experience

At Western Connecticut State University (WCSU), our first lab expansion involved many individuals from the Dean to the Chair to University computing to maintenance, purchasing, and accounts payable to name a few. The second expansion involved the President, purchasing, multiple assistants and secretaries, and university computing technicians as well as several faculty members. Currently, Phase 3 of this expansion project will result from a federal nursing initiative (US Department of Education—FIPSE P116Z080237, 2008) negotiated by the University Provost, and we will need many departments' help to renovate a space and to set up and maintain a lab. With a drastic increase in enrollment, expanding access to all levels of simulation is the primary goal. Having one or two people leading the way who have good relationships with all departments will facilitate the progress of the project, but an entire team working together during the implementation helps. Resources needed include work with Laerdal Create-a-Lab and the university architect developing the final layout. Many times, there is no time for new building, so making the most of the space you have, using fresh paint and minor renovations such as removing old cabinets, replacing countertops, and rewiring for equipment with diligence and hard work is best when time is of the essence. Often, labs will need to be set up during times when classes are not in session, such as the summer months. Although having a vision is crucial, be open to other ideas to get what is needed, even if it may look very different from the initial picture in your mind.

Dollars, Donations, and Finances

Funding new resource centers and expansion projects is costly and challenging. Most facilities have written multiple grants meeting with various successes and failures. Securing money from many sources is often necessary. It may take several months to years to secure adequate funding. In the case of WCSU, our simulation journey began to take shape after 2 years of grant writing. Three entities came together to finance the first HPS: the Vice President of Academic Affairs; the Dean's office; and the Director of University Computing, whose generosity provided the bulk of the money. Within 2 years, a new simulator and space were needed to provide more access to simulation. The timing was perfect, because a new science building on campus left the old building empty. With the backing of the University President, a five-room astronomy suite was designated as the new lab, and with cleaning, renovation, and electrical work, the space was made useable for us. Because the new science building was being finished, we had contractors on campus doing other work, so they were able to readily help with our renovations. In addition, another grant came in that year from which funds for equipment were secured. The lab was ready for the fall semester.

There has been much more work to do to upgrade the lab over time, but the space is an excellent area for an assessment lab, a simulation room, a seminar room, a pediatric lab, a classroom space with Internet access, and a resource room.

Individual faculty members have secured small grants for simulation projects, with funds for equipment embedded in the grant. This money was used to set up individual stations for each HPS. A crash cart or treatment cart works best to store the equipment needed for simulations. Each high-fidelity HPS began by residing in a hospital bed. These beds made it difficult to move the HPS. Stretchers work best to make the HPS movable. Some faculty have taken the HPS "on the road" by using wheelchairs. There are anecdotal reports that one HPS made it to graduation and made a speech! The more movable, the better for taking to class and doing mock codes in interesting places. Hospitals may donate minimally broken stretchers that are too dangerous for patients but are fine for a HPS.

Faculty have also secured summer curriculum funds in order to have focused time for scenario writing and setup. In addition, faculty have used faculty funds to attend training conferences, obtain time release for research studies using the new simulation equipment, and encourage faculty to get outside training. In addition, it was necessary to train the university technology staff to help with upgrades and troubleshooting.

Of course, the best-case scenario is when a very large grant or donation is secured to cover all aspects of a learning resource center.

Diana and Suzanne's Story: Fairfield University School of Nursing's Experience

For Fairfield University School of Nursing, the vision for the integration of simulation-focused learning developed over time and required support from a variety of individuals and groups. As is sometimes the case where the stars align and all the right pieces fall into place, we were fortunate to have that happen for us. In early 2005, there was a decentralizing of the development office at the university, which led to the School of Nursing receiving a designated development officer—the foundation relation officer. At about the same time, a nursing student graduated after working her senior year in the nursing lab and at the pinning ceremony handed the dean a check for $40,000 to purchase a HPS. Finally, a friend of the School of Nursing set up a Distinguished Lecturer Series and challenged the school to "plan for its future." The direct relationship with the development office in addition to the formation of the Distinguished Lecturer Series led to the formation of a School of Nursing Advisory Board (Appel, Campbell, Novotny, & Lynch, 2007). Nursing faculty worked on a vision and project plan for the Learning Resource Center, with the core of the project being to recognize the gaps in present nursing education and the benefits of simulation-focused pedagogy.

Administrative support from the Academic Vice President, Dean of the School of Nursing, and Foundation Relations Officer led to the development of the 4-year "Learning Resource Center Project," with Suzanne as the Project

Director and Diana as the Director of the Learning Resource Center. Diana's role was key to the integration of the project as well as nursing faculty input and enthusiasm. A university-wide committee was formed to get feedback and gather ideas in all areas, including upgrading classrooms, addition of new technology, purchasing simulation equipment, education of faculty and students in the use of the new equipment, the use of students for role-playing during scenarios, health communication specialists input for development of scenarios, and interdisciplinary guidance. Key to this vision was a plan specific to faculty development for this paradigm shift. The faculty development aspect will be discussed further in chapter 4.

In addition, the university was going through changes with a new President after 25 years as well as the development of the Center for Academic Excellence. The center provided university-wide support to promote the development of best practices in the Scholarship of Teaching and Learning. Faculty and staff, including media and informational technology, provided support and buy-in for the new project. In less than 3 years, the School of Nursing Advisory Board raised $1.06 million for the 4-year Learning Resource Center project.

From the project's initial conception in 2005, the facility renovation was completed in the summer of 2006. Two simulation rooms were created with control from a central, double-sided mirrored room that was placed in between them. Although present on the second floor of the School of Nursing, these classrooms originally held 30 students and were used by the whole university. This project converted them into specialty areas (an intensive care and an operating room) for simulation-only use exclusively by the School of Nursing. In addition, the three major classrooms in the School of Nursing were renovated with state-of-the-art technology, wireless systems, and faculty consoles with computer, LCD projector, DVD, and VCR capabilities. Write-on boards replace the blackboards and bulletin boards, and the computers have starboard technology for use during class. Both classrooms on the second floor are remotely connected to the simulation rooms so that larger groups of students can observe their classmates interacting during a scenario in one of the simulation rooms. Also, DVD recording of scenario implementation is feasible. The initial one-room lab was enhanced with LCD screens and computer technology; new cabinets and counters; and new furniture, including portable, stackable chairs and tables.

Originally, a small computer lab sat connected to the back of the major one-room lab. Over recent years, fewer and fewer students are using the computer lab, as many students bring their own laptops to the university, and many have access to desktop computers in their dorms. Due to the decrease in student traffic in the computer lab, we decided to convert this room into more usable space. It was converted into two separate areas by dividing the room with tall storage cabinets; on one side of the partition is a home care room, and on the other is a women's health room. With a recent state grant from the Connecticut Health and Education Facilities Authority (CHEFA) (2007), the women's health room has been expanded to include a labor and delivery staging area complete with an infant warmer, neonatal intensive care area with isolette, and a human infant simulator. In addition, acquisition of infant, child, and adult medium-fidelity technology has expanded the simulation possibilities for many specialty areas.

Finally, the largest classroom (an auditorium that seats 120 students) was equipped with the capability to record the class with live streaming of the audio, video, and PowerPoint slides available on the Internet. It has been used to teach students a nursing course while studying abroad, to prerecord a nursing course if a faculty member was at a conference, and to work with faculty abroad by presenting and sharing content. This technology would also work well to hold national and/or international workshops, such as simulation-building cases for more global and world health issues.

Although the rooms are in place and the equipment is being added on a year-to-year basis as the funds become available, the integration aspect of the project continues. Expecting faculty to "make the switch" to use a simulation-based pedagogy overnight is unrealistic, and we have found that with simple steps, such as having the technology available in the classroom, many are experimenting and making changes as they go. In general, most faculty have attended simulation workshops, begun to learn about the development of scenarios specific to their courses and content, and enjoyed the challenges of integrating simulation into their classes. Some significant questions have arisen and will be discussed in chapter 26. In addition, as the project director and lab director, we have found our roles to include supporting faculty in the development and running of their scenarios, being the HPS controller, or a role-player in the acting of the scenario as well as being ready at a moment's notice to problem solve the technology issues that arise. We have been most fortunate in the support from our media and IT teams, school and university administration, and not surprisingly, from the enthusiasm and excitement we recognize in students and colleagues as they learn about and use this simulation-focused pedagogy.

Over the last few years, federal and state entities have built large simulation centers with large budgets for equipment with the best intentions. However, not all faculty had enough simulation experience to be able to make the labs functional. They may have been thrown into the simulation whirlwind without any idea of what to buy or how to set up the simulation experiences, which can be a frustrating and intimidating situation. Chapters 21 and 22 provide a description of a large simulation center and how it was created to accommodate nursing students at various stages, including capstone simulation scenarios and interdisciplinary training.

Maintenance and Updating/Upgrading: Challenge of Continuous Funding

Of course, the good news is that simulation within a learning resource center can quickly become a well-used learning tool. This technology is often sought after by students picking colleges, matriculated students needing practice, and remediation and community agencies interested in simulation for staff training and professional development. The bad news is that even the best-made HPS will need occasional maintenance and upgrading. When planning a learning resource center with simulation, it is wise to plan for the technology help you will need to maintain the HPS. At WCSU, a few staff in the University Computing Department were interested, intrigued, and therefore very helpful whenever a technology issue arose. However, with our level of simulation expanding to what will be four high-fidelity HPS, University Computing is currently working to hire a nursing department technologist who will be responsible for all the technology. Many programs have talented lab assistants who are very helpful with the simulation but need technology help when it comes to upgrades and maintenance. I (Daley) have been known to say repeatedly, "I have my PhD in nursing, not computers!" That being said, I have enjoyed the challenge of learning the technologic aspect of simulation, but not all faculty share my enthusiasm. In addition, there are the challenges of ordering replacement supplies and the inevitable crash of one of the HPS who drowns in a simulated blood transfusion that springs a leak or a rouge IV that infuses into the bed and not the HPS. In those cases, and to address the inevitable technology issues, purchasing a maintenance plan and extended warranties and securing replacement HPSs is wise. Most simulator companies will have those options available at purchase. Funding those yearly costs can be a challenge and should be planned for when building and planning to maintain a learning resource center. Ideally, as is true at WCSU, our *very* generous Director of University Computing picks up those costs every year.

At Fairfield University, maintenance and warranty plans have been purchased. One of the unanticipated extra expenses had to do with rewiring for the new HPS model. Initially, the HPS was wired to connect to the control room so that a microphone in that room could switch back and forth and the instructor's voice could come from the room (with directions for students) or from the HPS (with responses from the patient to the student's questions). With the advent of new technology that directly connected the HPS to a touch screen monitor, rewiring was necessary and has caused many headaches. Even newer HPS will incorporate wireless technology, although with the concrete building in our 1970s nursing building, it is possible that wireless technology may not work from the control room to the simulation rooms. Some of these expenses are just not easily anticipated, and future planning for the inevitable is prudent.

The newer grants being processed and funded at Fairfield University include these expenses for IT support, lab support to run the scenarios, and technology upgrades. This adds additional administrative work to the faculty receiving the grants and needs to be carefully considered in their workload and future assignments. Other challenges include changes that occur at the university level, including but not restricted to changes in the course management system vendors, incorporation of university-wide portfolios as the portals to student learning, and continuous upgrading of classroom and faculty technologies (e.g., computers) to keep pace with the technologic advancements. Sometimes, learning to work with what you have, recognizing its potential, and visualizing how it fits in your curriculum is key, without thinking you have to have the newest and the most up-to-date materials. Purchasing the newest things on the market is a risky and time-consuming endeavor (see Table 3.1).

3.1 Key Points for Consideration in Building/Renovating Simulation Labs

	Fairfield University	Western Connecticut State University
Funding Sources	Private funds State funds—specific grants Applied for federal funds	Multiple grants from university, state, and federal funds
Initial Conceptualization	Conceptualized and funded first, grand wish list compiled, and consultant used for lab layout initially	Conceptualized first, then several rounds of small funding
Acquiring Physical Space	*Phase I:* Planned renovation of classroom space into large simulation area. Reclaimed areas within the School of Nursing. Includes advanced nursing care/ICU equipment and an OR area. Also, designation of existing lab space to simulation space specific for ICU, obstetrics, and home health. Basic upgrades to all spaces, including paint, window treatments, and lighting. *Phase II:* Expansion of obstetric facilities to include labor and delivery, postpartum, newborn nursery, and neonatal ICU with state grant funds (CHEFA, 2007). *Phase III:* Upgrading of OR area for nurse anesthetist student use with federal grant funds.	*Phase I:* Began with a small simulation area designated in existing lab. *Phase II:* Five-room suite space acquisition, room-by-room renovations, and flexible use of space. Addition of resource rooms over time to each area. *Phase III:* Designed and renovated area on another campus with separate simulation room adjacent to a new traditional lab. *Phase IV:* New space acquired and renovated for advanced nursing care/ICU (US Department of Education—FIPSE P116Z080237, 2008).
Technology	Three high-fidelity HPS: one medium-fidelity obstetric HPS; one each medium-fidelity adult, child, and infant HPS; and static task trainers Large state-of-the-art controller room that can view both simulation rooms with video, audio, and projection capabilities. Large auditorium with Media-Site Live capability for live-streaming audio/video of classes and simulations	Four high-fidelity HPS; one medium-fidelity pediatric simulator, three static mannequins and task trainers One scenario controller station. PDA scenario controllers on all other HPS
Actual Facility Space	All simulation equipment housed in one building in adjacent rooms	Simulation facilities housed in three separate buildings and on two campuses
Personnel	Diana Mager, Director. Robin Kanarek Learning Resource Center. Suzanne Hetzel Campbell, Project Director. Work-study students staff the lab during semesters for student practice. Instructors run own scenarios with assistance from directors, other faculty, and each other. Acquiring a part-time technology assistant and lab assistant as part of state grant for fiscal year 2008–2009.	No lab assistant. Simulations run by individual instructors. Staffed with work-study students who open the lab for student practice. Load credit for maintaining lab and resources given to Learning Resources Committee chair or faculty who provide lab instruction and remediation. Acquiring a technology assistant for maintaining simulators in fall 2008.

Continuous Funding	The initial vision of the project outlined a 4-year time line, and a budget was developed to incorporate all aspects: building and classroom renovation, equipment purchasing, faculty development, and assessment and evaluation. Several grant applications have been submitted to assist with funding through grants. The Associate Dean of Public Health and Entrepreneurial Initiatives is also the assistant director of this project and is creating opportunities for unique and innovative funding (see chapter 25).	Information Technology Department of the university partially funded initial purchase of first HPS. Going forward, the Information Technology Department has taken on responsibility of maintaining maintenance and warranty contracts, supervision of the computers and computer technology necessary to run simulators, and provide technology assistance as needed.
Faculty Development	HPS training and workshops provided by HPS company: faculty attendance and presentation at national and regional simulation and education conferences funded through faculty development funds. Faculty workshops for scenario writing, electronic medical record integration, and curriculum redesign held on campus throughout the semester. Small stipend for faculty participation. Individual Faculty Learning Community in place in 2007–2008, with subsequent course redesign and project development (see chapter 4). Individualized training as needed. Support from University Center for Academic Excellence. Full day-and-a-half retreat planned for fall 2008 for curriculum development and technology integration for all School of Nursing faculty.	HPS training and workshops provided by HPS company: individualized faculty to faculty training and small group as needed. New faculty training as requested by the Learning Resources Committee chair and current high-level faculty users. Faculty use faculty development and travel funds to attend training and seminars on simulation.
Assessment and Evaluation	Five-year assessment plan in place. Outside assessment team hired, university assessment director involved, baseline data gathered on all four cohorts of students in year 1 (2007–2008) in the form of surveys, focus groups, and student work and artifacts (including reflections). Other methods for program assessment will include the following: ERI scores on RN-Assess tests, NCLEX pass rates, alumni survey data, and employer survey data as well as university-wide assessment tests. More specifically for individual class projects, faculty are assessing student work and reflection to determine effects of the new teaching paradigm.	Currently in year 1 of full assessment plan after a 3-year development phase. The evaluation of simulation is embedded throughout the curriculum by documenting the overall program outcomes. Continued evaluation of the effects of simulation will be carried out by examining: NCLEX pass rates, pre- and post testing in the capstone course, and graduate and employer surveys. We feel strongly that simulation helps us to address all program outcomes, specifically: thinking critically, communicating effectively, and performing nursing interventions appropriate to the practice role.

ICU, intensive care unit; OR, operating room; HPS, human patient simulator; PDA, personal digital assistant; ERI, Educational Research Inc.; RN, registered nurse; NCLEX, National Council Licensure Examination

Conclusion

We recognize the variety of programs, needs, and resources for each school of nursing. The complex factors of university strategic plans and missions, administrative support, outside funding opportunities, and the like are beyond the breadth and depth of this book. However, we hope that through sharing our stories, we have given you some insight into potential problems that may arise as well as ways to best meet the challenges associated with this paradigm shift. The other authors have shared their stories throughout this book, about how they are using simulation, the type of environment, and what needs specific to their disciplines are most helpful for the successful integration of simulation.

Change is never easy, and finding a champion to lead faculty, students, administration, and staff down this path makes a big difference in how it is perceived and how likely it is to succeed. The take-home message is this: Persist, go slowly, think outside the box, and garnish the support of those around you to create a vision of how things will work best for you, your faculty, your university, and your students. But most importantly, *have fun!* Share your stories. Laugh, learn, and embrace the process. The potential for growth is limitless. Good luck!

References

Appel, N., Campbell, S. H., Lynch, N., & Novotny, J. (2007). Creating effective advisory boards for schools of nursing. *Journal of Professional Nursing, 23*(6), 343–350.

Connecticut Health and Education Facilities Authority (CHEFA). (2007). CHEFA grant for $99,999.00 women's health simulation expansion project. Pilot team: Suzanne Campbell (P.I.), Diana DeBartolomeo Mager (Co-P.I.), Phil Greiner, Sheila Grossman, and Alison Kris.

U.S. Department of Education—FIPSE P116Z080237. (2008). CSUS Initiative to Improve the Capacity and Preparation of the Nursing Workforce. Karen Daley & Debra LaJoie (Co-Project Directors). $130,000 for expansion of simulation for retention/remediation and scholarships.

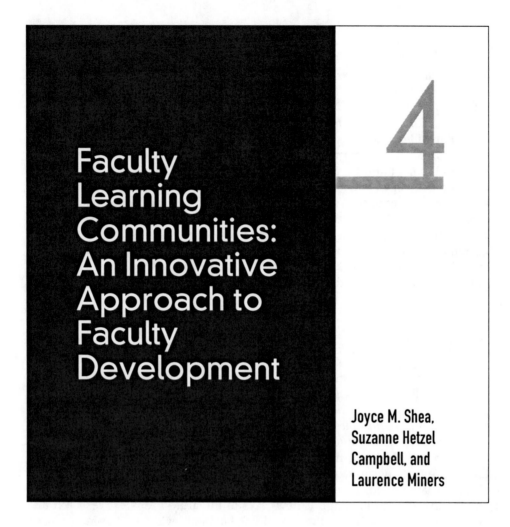

Faculty Learning Communities: An Innovative Approach to Faculty Development

Joyce M. Shea,
Suzanne Hetzel
Campbell, and
Laurence Miners

The demands for meeting the needs of 21st-century students, especially in the health professions, are increasing exponentially. One form of technology, simulation, has been recognized as a valuable tool for the development of critical thinking and clinical competence in nursing students (Chau, Chang, Lee, Ip, Lee, & Wootton, 2001; Jeffries, 2005; Nehring, Lashley, & Ellis, 2002; Peteani, 2004; Rauen, 2001). While students tend to favor the use of simulation in teaching (Feingold, Calaluce, & Kallen, 2004), faculty can be resistant to this complex teaching methodology (Nehring & Lashley, 2004). Because of this, and the high costs associated with the use of patient simulators in nursing education (Harlow & Sportsman, 2007; Metcalfe, Hall, & Carpenter, 2007), care must be taken in the planning, implementation, and evaluation of simulation-based programs.

As mentioned in chapter 3, faculty buy-in is of the utmost importance in a successful integration of simulation and technology into the nursing curriculum. With all the advances in education and technology, nursing faculty can feel overwhelmed with the increasing expectations. They need time to integrate these new teaching tools and receive assistance with the actual process. What better method than in a group of peers with dedicated time to explore the possibilities and actually integrate new tools into the courses they are teaching?

Traditionally, faculty who take on this type of initiative may at best receive course release time to revise a course on their own. Usually, it is another "expected addition" to the faculty role. The equipment is purchased, a lab director oversees, and faculty are expected to work this out.

To provide optimum student learning experiences, changes in educational practices need to be incorporated with pedagogic principles, which in turn guide the development and implementation of simulation activities and the integration of technology (Jeffries, 2005). Faculty need to be given the opportunity to reflect on connections between simulation and (1) their individual teaching philosophy and (2) the attainment of student competency in core areas. One such opportunity for reflection occurred in our School of Nursing Faculty Learning Community (FLC), a small group of faculty who made a yearlong commitment to meet for scheduled biweekly meetings to participate in active dialogue regarding enhancing faculty competency in teaching/learning pedagogy and technology (Cox, 2004a, p. 8).

One School's Story

Fairfield University is a small, private, Jesuit institution that was established in 1942 as an all-male school. In 1970, it became co-educational and welcomed its first students into the School of Nursing. The mission of Fairfield University is to develop the *creative intellectual potential* of its students and to foster in them: ethical and religious values, a sense of social responsibility, truth, and justice. The School of Nursing curriculum reflects this mission through a small, close-knit academic environment with class sizes of approximately 30 students per class, the large majority being residential students, which adds to the sense of community. Always looking for new ways to integrate the latest research and clinical practice guidelines, the school has taken an evidence-based approach to nursing, such as through the use of simulation pedagogy. Over 50 clinical agencies from hospitals to community-based organizations expose students to a wide variety of experiences. Simulation increases opportunities for faculty to provide consistent clinical experiences for students as well as to help them understand and prepare for the context of rapid technologic, demographic, and health care system changes.

The faculty role has evolved beyond a "talking head" providing didactic content from behind a lectern. Today's students demand interactive formats that engage and excite them. In this paradigm shift, faculty become mentors and focus on role-modeling and facilitating diverse experiences in a safe environment. Nursing faculty seem to be comfortable in this role with their years of clinical education. However, getting students to be more engaged in the learning process and requiring a level of preparation prior to coming to class continues to be a challenge. In addition, the costs of diverse technologies and methods and initial and maintenance costs as well as support and staff development can be considerable. Getting back to faculty buy-in for the process—is there any easy way?

In chapter 3, the experience of Fairfield University's School of Nursing related to the creation of the vision for a learning resource center was described. The funds set aside specifically for faculty development were used for a variety of opportunities, including workshop and conference attendance, retreats, mentoring consultants, and course release for innovative course development. When the director of the Center of Academic Excellence (CAE) met with the project director and Learning Resource Center committee, a budget and plan for 4-year project development was put into place. The rest of this chapter will describe this plan as seven nursing faculty were supported to participate in the yearlong School of Nursing FLC.

Relationship to University Initiatives

In July 2004, Fairfield University hired a new president, and in his inaugural address, Reverend Jeffrey P. von Arx, S. J., outlined a new vision for the university. He called for the university "to become recognized for leadership in producing graduates whose lives reflect personal integration, competence in multicultural understanding, and a commitment to professional responsibility" (von Arx, *Learning and integrity: A strategic vision for Fairfield University,* intercampus communication, 2005). During the first 18 months of his administration, the university community formulated a new 10-year strategic plan for the university. There are three main cornerstones of the plan: the integration of the core curriculum, the integration of living and learning, and the integration of Jesuit values in graduate and professional education. The creation of the Learning Resource Center in the School of Nursing in 2006, as well as the school's subsequent efforts to create a more integrated and holistic curriculum, fit perfectly in the university's strategic plan.

As part of the effort to integrate the core curriculum, both with courses in a student's major and with Fairfield's Jesuit identity, the CAE began a series of FLCs. These communities were created around themes and sought to bring together faculty members who wanted to learn more about integrated teaching and were interested in changing pedagogy.

The CAE is Fairfield's faculty resource center and endeavors to improve student learning by fostering faculty inquiry into the learning process. The notion of academic excellence includes excellence in pedagogy; excellence in scholarship; and excellence in faculty–student relations in the classroom, laboratory, or anywhere learning occurs. The CAE provides a central place on campus dedicated to support the development and promulgation of the best in new pedagogical methods and the expansion of faculty–student research opportunities.

Overview of Faculty Learning Communities

The FLC initiative at Fairfield University is modeled after the FLC program started by Dr. Milton Cox at Miami University in Ohio in the late 1970s. At Miami, an FLC is defined as "a cross-disciplinary faculty and staff group of six to fifteen members or more (eight to twelve members is the recommended size) engaging in an active, collaborative, yearlong program with a curriculum about enhancing teaching and learning" (Cox, 2004b, Section 1B). There are two main organizational structures of FLCs: topic-based groups that devote their attention to a specific pedagogically related topic (e.g., diversity, spirituality, environment), representing approximately three-quarters of FLCs nationwide; and cohort-based

FLCs (e.g., untenured faculty, mid-career faculty, department chairs). FLCs are typically comprised of a heterogeneous mix of participants. For the needs of the School of Nursing, the FLC came about as a result of a topic-based need (integrating simulation) and a cohort-based need (to enhance the cohesiveness of the curriculum across the nursing program). For this school-specific FLC, heterogeneity was represented by the participants' different research specialties and teaching areas as well as the inclusion of the lab director, traditionally a staff rather than a faculty position. The nursing FLC also included a mix of untenured, mid-career, and senior-level faculty members.

The collaboration between the School of Nursing and the CAE started well before the initiation of the FLC program. Early on, the directors of the Learning Resource Center, the CAE, and others met to discuss the creation of the Center and the redesign of the nursing curriculum. The CAE was part of the initiative that launched and explained the goals of the project to faculty members in the School of Nursing. The School's initiative was linked to the university's strategic plan, and the FLC model was proposed to the faculty. All members were invited to apply, and the resulting FLC included half of the full-time faculty in the School of Nursing.

The nursing FLC was run in tandem with four other FLCs, and there was a concerted attempt to create bridges across the five programs. The CAE spent a year designing the program and attempted, as much as the individual communities desired, to follow a common model of facilitation. Participants reacted favorably to the opening workshop, the mid-year seminar, and the closing session, in which all groups were present. The four other university FLCs focused on environment studies, international studies, teaching to diversity, and teaching with technology.

Overall, the goals of the FLC program at Fairfield mirrored closely those outlined by Cox (2004b) at Miami University:

(1) Build university-wide community through teaching and learning, creating a learning organization, (2) increase faculty interest in undergraduate teaching and learning, (3) increase the rewards for and prestige of excellent teaching, (4) investigate and incorporate ways that diversity can enhance teaching and learning, (5) nourish scholarly teaching and the scholarship of teaching and its application to student learning, (6) broaden the evaluation of teaching, (7) encourage and motivate new approaches to teaching and learning, (8) create an awareness of the complexity of teaching and learning, (9) increase faculty collaboration across disciplines, (10) increase civic responsibility and interest in institution-wide perspectives, (11) broaden the assessment of student learning, and (12) encourage reflection about liberal education and coherence of learning across disciplines. (Section 3.1)

How the Nursing Faculty Learning Community Functioned

FLCs differ from faculty committees in some fundamental ways. Most obvious is the emphasis on forming community. Decisions are usually made by consensus rather than votes, and a sincere effort is made to accommodate dissenting opinions. The facilitator works to make sure all voices are heard. Listening and thoughtful reflection are encouraged; long position-entrenching monologues are discouraged. The facilitator helps to guide the community but does not set the agenda; rather, he or she helps to guide the group down the path (or agenda) that was mutually agreed on. The nursing FLC was facilitated by the director of the CAE, who is also a faculty member in the Economics Department. At the end of each meeting, time was set aside so that the group could reflect on what was being taken away from the meeting. Community members wrote these statements in private and then shared their writing with the group. This exercise led to deeper insights of the FLC experience and helped motivate people to share with their colleagues.

Conceptual and Practical Issues

Members of the School of Nursing FLC initially joined the group for the express purpose of integrating simulation into various courses across the curriculum. As the group began to meet, however, it became clear that the work needed to begin with an exploration and discussion about *why* simulation needed to be integrated and *how* we might best accomplish this for our curriculum. The result was a search for an appropriate conceptual basis for the use of simulation and recognition of the need to clarify the stated goals of the nursing curriculum. In effect, the Nursing FLC became a *think tank* for the identification of specific program outcomes and consideration of simulation as one mechanism for reaching those outcomes.

Early discussion focused on such broad-based phenomena as the shift in nursing education to student-centered learning objectives (Iwasiw, Goldenberg, & Andrusyszyn, 2005) and pedagogical transformation in higher education to incorporate more social-emotional and reflective-type learning (Institute of Noetic Sciences, 2007). The concept of *Emotional Intelligence* was explored for its implications in the areas of nursing education (Freshwater & Stickley, 2004), nursing practice (Kooker, Shoultz, & Codier, 2007), and nursing leadership (Herbert & Edgar, 2004). Simulation seemed to be an especially useful tool to help students begin to develop a balance between the rational and emotional minds and to utilize reflective learning that moves them beyond the level of abstract or practical knowledge. Ultimately, discussions on self-reflection brought members of the FLC to readings involving the concept of *mindfulness,* or consciousness and being present in the moment, which plays a key role in the psychological well-being of individuals (Brown & Ryan, 2003) and impacts the ability of the nursing student to assess and demonstrate clinical reasoning skills. The final search for an appropriate conceptual basis for the integration of simulation across the curriculum resulted in the discovery of the process of integrated learning as described by Siegel (2007). Group members agreed on the relevance of Siegel's neurobiologic theory of learning, which is based on the integration of right- and left brain function and his description of links to reflective thinking. The theory recognizes the importance of combining concrete memorization with experiential learning and describes how both contribute to the development of new neural pathways or networks in the brain and an increase in what would be considered significant learning. Simulation, in all its variations, seems to be a perfect mechanism for promoting cognitive (i.e., critical thinking) and metacognitive (i.e., reflective thinking) skills, and the right- and left brain functioning, of nursing students.

The FLC structure also allowed the nursing faculty to deal with a number of practical issues that arose during its meetings. Members were able to define and refine the role that technology might play in various courses throughout the nursing curriculum. For example, courses such as Critical Care Nursing had an obvious need to rely on complex technology and high-fidelity simulators as part of their content and assignments, while courses such as Mental Health Nursing began to carve out a role for simulations using human actors to bring clinical situations and learning to life. While all FLC members became more comfortable with the notion of technology and simulation through their work in the group, they also recognized the need to be available to those nursing faculty who had not participated in the FLC to help foster their level of comfort with simulation. Time was also spent in the FLC meetings discussing issues such as planning for ongoing support (financial and otherwise) for the implementation of a simulation-focused pedagogy—both from within and outside the School of Nursing—and for the potential role of simulation in program assessment and the overall accreditation process. Suggestions were made and plans were developed to use simulation to provide documentation of individual student competencies and progress toward program goals and national benchmarks.

Outcomes of the School of Nursing Faculty Learning Community

The most tangible outcome for the members of the Nursing FLC were the individual projects they developed for specific courses. These projects involved students in courses that ranged from undergraduate to graduate levels and in all specialty areas. Three of these projects are described here in detail.

For the Nursing Care of Women and Children, 21 junior students enhanced their reflective learning in a number of ways: via reflective logs after clinical experiences; using interactive learning experiences, including videos of nurse–patient interactions; specific assessments; role-playing for simulated scenarios; and presentation of case studies. Increases in student self-confidence were measured using pre- and post-course assessments. Information was also collected on mindfulness and student perceptions of learning strategies that enhanced their reflective learning. In addition, a cumulative self-reflection was collected in document form on their growth, challenges, and future goals in four areas: personal growth, clinical growth, communication skills, and professional behavior.

For a graduate nurse practitioner course, the goal was to increase student mindfulness to learning by incorporating active learning techniques with the use of case studies, application to student's prior clinical experience, and evidence-based guidelines for practice. Self-reflection with written logs, prescription writing, microsimulation, role-playing, and written case study analysis review were all used to integrate and enhance learning. Assessment of mindfulness and student perceptions of best learning strategies for reflective learning was evaluated at the beginning and end of the course.

Finally, an application to a lab course involved faculty focusing on the development of fundamental nursing skills by incorporating a critical thinking component into written situational dilemmas (similar to case studies but with a problem related to the skill being tested). Situations were worth 5 points, and instructor critique and comments were used to help students integrate and analyze their critical and reflective thinking. Evaluation consisted of student interviews to determine if the activity contributed to their learning in terms of enhancing reflective and critical thinking skills.

Overall, faculty who participated in the School of Nursing FLC felt that they had gained significant insight into how the right- and left brain work and learn, including the right brain's template for affect regulation and a healthy sense of self. The concept of mindfulness was explored in detail, and many faculty took pre- and postmeasures of student mindfulness at the start and end of their semester classes. Readings from the scholarship of teaching and learning, nursing education, and clinical skill development also contributed to faculty growth.

These readings and discussions promoted reflection on teaching practices and a focus on case study writing and reflective learning. Faculty shared novel classroom techniques, and this encouraged others to experiment, such as with simple or complex simulation scenarios and/or various styles of reflection. In addition, faculty examined the nursing curriculum with a goal of looking for ways to improve critical thinking in students. Faculty felt that the work of the FLC was infused into simulation-based learning and promoted reflection on teaching practices.

Comments from School of Nursing FLC members included that they felt the group provided time and space for "collaboration/connection with colleagues" and "collegiality, camaraderie, trust, honesty"; and they felt they had a "safe, comfortable place to experiment with new ideas to enhance teaching/learning"; the time itself was "special, sacred time"; and the mantra of all was "We will always be a group!" Faculty felt reinforced that no matter how long they had been teaching, there were vulnerabilities and struggles experienced by all. Finally, the support of the CAE was superb; FLC members felt that the CAE was responsive to their needs with provision of wonderful resources (such as books, speakers, conference support) and that the facilitator was very receptive to the group's requests.

In addition, other tangible outcomes included the following: state grant funding from CHEFA for the Women's Health Simulation project mentioned in chapter 3, with a total of $99,999, including both equipment and lab support in the form of information technology and lab assistants; and national and international conference presentations, including one focusing on FLCs and another on the use of case studies. Finally, the work by the individual School of Nursing FLC members resulted in chapters for this book as well as changes to courses and evaluation of student learning.

Future Direction

The FLC afforded us a vehicle by which we developed a much more comprehensive and visionary approach to the integration of simulation. It gave us the means not only to implement specific strategies but to assess the impact on outcomes such as the following:

- *Increased continuity of classroom and clinical experiences:* With this as a long-term goal, our involvement in the FLC allowed much more comprehensive and thoughtful reflection on how the changes in classroom pedagogy affect clinical experiences of students.
- *The effect of technology:* Technology is seen not just as a vehicle for learning (e.g., simulation) but as a mechanism for a more comprehensive and visionary approach to the integration of an interactive learning environment. It also gives us the means not only to implement the strategies but also to assess the impact on these outcomes:
  - Integration of pedagogy across the curriculum
  - Enhanced student learning
  - Expertise integrating technology into clinical practice
  - Increased critical and reflective thinking in all settings

In conclusion, as a group, we felt better prepared to continue to develop and evaluate overall program goals and objectives. We will continue to reflect as a faculty on what we want to accomplish and how we might accomplish it through the use of simulation (or varied learning methods). There has been talk of "keeping in touch," and, as the overall School of Nursing faculty is small (almost half of the full-time faculty were part of this group), it seems feasible that an informal FLC might be organized. During the next academic year (2008–2009), another member of the nursing faculty is joining a new university FLC focusing on spirituality in education. We look forward to hearing what she learns as she will undoubtedly benefit from the broadened experience and contact with colleagues across the university. The School of Nursing FLC also shared its "graduation presentation" with the entire School of Nursing and found that discussions at faculty and curriculum meetings as well as workshops on assessment and simulation often reflected some aspect of the work of the group. All in all, the FLC experience was a success in allowing members to reflect, plan, and implement efforts to integrate simulation and assess its impact throughout the nursing curriculum.

References

Brown, K. W., & Ryan, R. M. (2003). The benefits of being present: Mindfulness and its role in psychological well-being. *Journal of Personality and Social Psychology, 84,* 822–848.

Chau, J. P. C., Chang, A. M., Lee, I. F. K., Ip, W. Y., Lee, D. T. F., & Wootton, Y. (2001). Effects of using videotaped vignettes on enhancing students' critical thinking ability in a baccalaureate nursing programme. *Journal of Advanced Nursing, 36,* 112–119.

Cox, M. D. (2004a). Introduction to faculty learning communities. *New Directions for Teaching and Learning, 97,* 5–23.

Cox, M. D. (2004b). *Faculty learning community program director's handbook and facilitator's handbook FIPSE project* (2nd ed.). Miami, FL: Miami University.

Feingold, C. E., Calaluce, M., & Kallen, M. (2004). Computerized patient model and simulated clinical experiences: Evaluation with baccalaureate nursing students. *Journal of Nursing Education, 43,* 156–163.

Freshwater, D., & Stickley, T. (2004). The heart of the art: Emotional intelligence in nurse education. *Nursing Inquiry, 11,* 91–98.

Harlow, K. C., & Sportsman, S. (2007). An economic analysis of patient simulators for clinical training in nursing education. *Nursing Economic$, 25*, 24–29.

Herbert, R., & Edgar, L. (2004). Emotional intelligence: A primal dimension of nursing leadership? *Nursing Leadership, 17*, 56–63.

Institute of Noetic Sciences. (2007). Education: Inward pedagogy. In *The 2007 shift report. Evidence of a world transforming* (pp. 57–61). Petaluma, CA: Author.

Iwasiw, C. L., Goldenberg, D., & Andrusyszyn, M. (2005). Extending the evidence base for nursing education. *International Journal of Nursing Education Scholarship, 2*(1), 1–3.

Jeffries, P. R. (2005). A framework for designing, implementing, and evaluating simulations used as teaching strategies in nursing. *Nursing Education Perspectives, 26*, 96–103.

Kooker, B. M., Shoultz, J., & Codier, E. E. (2006). Identifying emotional intelligence in professional nursing practice. *Journal of Professional Nursing, 23*, 30–36.

Metcalfe, S. E., Hall, V. P., & Carpenter, A. (2007). Promoting collaboration in nursing education: The development of a regional simulation laboratory. *Journal of Professional Nursing, 23*, 180–183.

Nehring, W. M., & Lashley, F. R. (2004). Current use and opinions regarding human patient simulators in nursing education: An international survey. *Nursing Education Perspectives, 25*, 244–248.

Nehring, W. M., Lashley, F. R., & Ellis, W. E. (2002). Critical incident nursing management using human patient simulators. *Nursing Education Perspectives, 23*, 128–132.

Peteani, L. A. (2004). Enhancing clinical practice and education with high-fidelity human patient simulators. *Nurse Educator, 29*, 25–30.

Rauen, C. A. (2001). Using simulation to teach critical thinking skills: You can't just throw the book at them. *Critical Care Nursing Clinics of North America, 13*, 93–103.

Seigel, D. (2007). *The mindful brain: Reflection and attunement in the cultivation of well-being*. New York: WW Norton & Company.

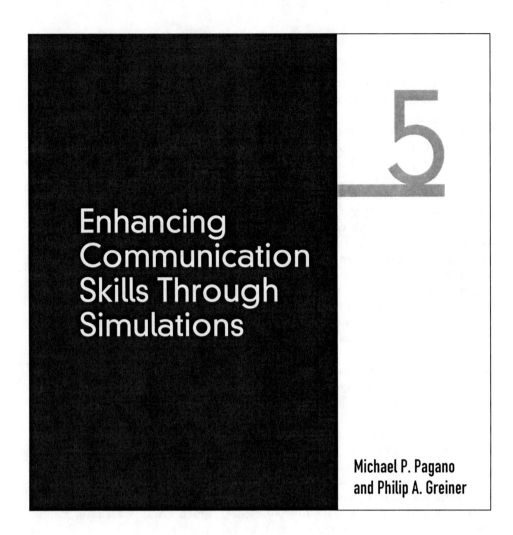

Enhancing Communication Skills Through Simulations

5

Michael P. Pagano
and Philip A. Greiner

Intrapersonal, Interpersonal, and Small Group Communication

Advances in technology have provided expanded opportunities in health care assessments and treatment options. However, technology is also expanding the abilities of nursing faculty to enhance the clinical training of their students. Simulations and the use of technologic advances like human patient simulators are excellent methods for assessing clinical skills prior to working at an actual patient's bedside. The added importance of this technology is that it can provide a wealth of information about a student's scientific and technical skills and at the same time allow faculty to evaluate and critique a student's health communication skills.

While the value of nurse–patient, nurse–peer, and nurse–team communication is well documented, the ability of nursing faculty to observe, assess, and direct their students' communication behaviors has been difficult (Arford, 2005; Leonard, Graham, & Bonacum, 2004). Direct observation of each student's communication in these diverse interactions has been difficult and almost impossible due to time constraints and the very nature of clinical practice and student–faculty ratios. Faculty cannot be in each patient's room while nursing students interact or always present when nurse–peer or nurse–team communication occurs. Therefore, in the past, the evaluation of those communication skills and behaviors were frequently assessed using third-party input and/or analyses of the student's task accomplishments and the student's self-appraisal of his or her performance.

Using simulations, nursing faculty have the ability to observe, assess, and provide feedback for student–patient, student–peer, and student–team communication in a clinical-type setting, with or without faculty being present. The advantages, from a health communication perspective, are multifaceted. Faculty can create simulations that focus on key clinical skills and related communication behaviors. During simulations, students can interact in a setting that mimics a clinical experience without fear of harming a patient and without faculty in the room but with a "patient" who can talk and provide feedback—both physiologically and interactively. In addition, the simulation can include other members of the health care team and/or the "patient's family members" to further enhance the learning opportunities.

This chapter will discuss how communication can be incorporated into the learning objectives and outcomes for simulations. The benefits of incorporating communication components into simulations for students, faculty, future patients, and peers will also be discussed.

The effectiveness of health communication generally depends on the success of intrapersonal communication (an individual's communication with herself or himself), interpersonal communication (communication between two individuals), and/or small group or team communication (between 3–20 people who share a common goal). While observation of communication is possible in traditional clinical nursing education, the evaluation of the communication is difficult, especially in interpersonal or small group situations. Evaluation requires direct observation and interaction, which takes time. Staffing limitations, and the settings themselves, make it hard to spend much time directly observing individuals in various settings. As well, research into the Hawthorne effect (Mayo, 1945; Shockley-Zalabak, 2006) has demonstrated the impact on an individual's communication when he or she is being directly observed.

With simulations, however, a faculty member can easily create scenarios that help to assess a student's critical thinking (intrapersonal communication); interpersonal communication with a patient, relative, or peer; or the student's group communication with team members. By "pseudo-covertly" (when something is known to the student but cameras and microphones are not intrusive in the setting, thus potentially reducing the Hawthorne effect) recording both the physiologic aspects of the scenario and the communication behaviors of the individuals, faculty can assess the interaction that occurs. In addition, faculty can also use the recordings as a tool to help enhance the communication effectiveness of the observed student and as training for other students (Washington University School of Medicine, 2006).

Furthermore, by allowing students to practice interpersonal communication in a "safe" setting, not in front of a sick or anxious person, concerned family members, or busy peers, nursing students can feel empowered to take on their new role and not risk saying or doing something that would harm a patient or embarrass themselves. The goal of such simulations is to encourage students to use interpersonal communication to build an interpersonal relationship with the patient, relatives, peers, and members of the team. Effective interpersonal relationships encourage trust among communicators and enhance information exchange and empowerment.

Similarly, by creating simulations that include peers and other actors as team members (doctors, technicians, dietitians, etc.), small group communication can be evaluated and enhanced. With the increasing emphasis on teamwork in health care, the importance of communication to group dynamics, leadership, group roles, and goal attainment are critical for nursing students. Consequently, the ability to develop simulations for various team settings (those in labor and delivery, the operating room, or running a code), provide excellent opportunities to assess and enhance students' small group behaviors and communication. It is this ability to create settings that illustrate and demonstrate a student's leadership and delegation skills that afford faculty a unique assessment tool.

Nonverbal Communication Assessment

Nonverbal communication is a key part of intrapersonal, interpersonal, and group communication. Research by Birdwhistell (1970), Mehrabian (1981), and Wood (2005) has shown that nonverbal behaviors are used by receivers in an interaction as more communicative of a message than verbal behaviors. For nursing students who are trying to concentrate on enhancing their clinical skills, it is often difficult to pay attention to nonverbal communication. Yet, research has shown that nonverbal communication is critically important to receivers. For example, a simulation that asks a student to take a patient's vital signs can certainly yield data about the student's ability to accurately obtain those numeric measures and proficiently use a blood pressure cuff and stethoscope. But perhaps as important an outcome for the simulation is the information observed about how the student used nonverbal behaviors and interpersonal communication to build the relationship that needs to be established with every patient. The simulation can help to identify if the student effectively used key nonverbal behaviors such as the following:

- Smiling (facial gesture) when greeting the patient
- Offering to shake hands (haptics, or touch)
- Making eye contact (gaze) when communicating
- Speaking clearly and in a loud enough voice to be easily heard (paralinguistic)

These nonverbal behaviors (facial gestures, haptics, gaze, and paralinguistic cues) are all important skills for enhancing interpersonal communication and relationships. Simulations then offer both faculty and students a chance to practice not only the clinical skills of measuring blood pressure, pulse, and respirations but also the interpersonal skills of building a relationship that will be critical when the nurse eventually wants to educate and empower patients in addition to gathering numeric clinical data.

Another way that simulations can help to increase student awareness of their nonverbal behaviors and their impact on their patients and others is by feedback from the patient, peer, relative, or team member in the simulation. For example, a nursing student comes to a simulation and says "Hello," then reaches for the patient's pulse. The patient or faculty could respond, "Who are you, and what are you doing?" This simple response would illustrate for the student that while he or she has a task to perform, it must be recognized that patients in this culture have very specific expectations regarding proxemics, the nonverbal communication of territoriality or personal space. Research by Hall (1959), Lyman and Scott, (1967), Rosenfeld and Civikly (1976), and Trenholm and Jensen (2008) has clearly demonstrated that Americans allow only intimates into their "personal space," which extends from 0 inches to 18 inches. So, when someone who is not an intimate uses haptics to invade a person's space, the person feels threatened. The nonverbal behaviors of trespassing in a patient's personal space, and touching him or her without permission, may have serious consequences to the establishment of an interpersonal relationship and to the effectiveness of interpersonal communication. An additional concern is the power dynamic that such an invasion of personal space conveys. Being a patient often shifts power from the patient to the provider. The assumption of intimacy and the student's nonverbal communication can be discussed in the debriefing.

It takes only seconds to explain the reason for the nursing student's visit and what he or she needs to do, but that verbal communication can comfort the patient by explaining the need for the nonverbal behaviors that follow. By appropriately using nonverbal and verbal behaviors to communicate his or her understanding of patients' rights to control what happens to their bodies, the nurse can communicate a desire to work not paternalistically but collaboratively with the patient.

Verbal Communication Assessment

Like nonverbal communication, verbal communication can be easily assessed, critiqued, and enhanced using simulations. In addition to clinical tasks, faculty can use scenarios to evaluate how students use language appropriate for the individuals in the simulation. For example, if a nursing student is asked to educate a patient and/or relatives about diabetes and administering insulin injections, the simulation could be evaluated on the nursing student's injection techniques: sterility, site location, withdrawing medication, and dosage delivered. However, just as important would be an assessment of the student's ability to choose words and phrases that are appropriate for the language skills and health literacy level of the patient and/or relatives. The simulation could help to reinforce the need for feedback, both nonverbal and verbal, in order to assess understanding and assimilation. Did the student look at the person while instructing to see if the patient and relatives were nodding in agreement or making facial expressions that indicate confusion? Did the student ask questions of the person being instructed about what the person heard and understood? Or perhaps a more effective approach, since it is less authoritarian, did the student ask the person to teach what was just discussed or shown? By asking the patient or relative to demonstrate what was learned, it is less of a quiz situation. All too often, communicators think that if no one asks questions, then everything has been understood, but in fact, people often do not ask questions, especially people from other cultures, because they do not understand what was being said and feel uncomfortable admitting it. So, a simulation can use feedback, or the lack of feedback, to help educate nursing students about using the appropriate level of health literacy in assessing the receiver's education and understanding of what is being communicated.

Simulations afford faculty the added opportunity to assess students' verbal communication based on a variety of contexts, or settings. Instead of having to go to a patient's bedside, the operating room, emergency department, labor and delivery, and the like, students can take on a role based on the context and scenario. Thus, a student's nursing communication can be assessed by his or her verbal skills in a setting that mimics a patient transfer and how information must be clearly communicated, using nursing vocabulary. In addition, medication reconciliation procedures can be assessed as well as the use of feedback and questioning. The difficulties of communicating information over a telephone, where nonverbal behaviors of receivers cannot be assessed, can be included in the context assessment. Each of these communication topics address Joint Commission on Accreditation of Healthcare Organizations and Institute of Medicine areas of concern for patient safety and quality of care (Aspden, Wolcott, Bootman, & Cronenwett, 2008, WHO Collaborating Centres for Patient Safety Solutions, 2007).

Furthermore, using various contexts for simulations, designed specifically to provide an opportunity for students to experience difficult situations and in a controlled environment, can be a very powerful learning experience. For example, creating simulations that involve emotional contexts (a dying patient and communication with him or her and/or the family or consoling or counseling the family of a seriously ill child) gives students a chance to feel the emotions of a situation but communicate in an environment that is supportive and reaffirming. In addition, simulations can be developed to mimic crisis settings or home care situations so that students experience the very different communication styles and behaviors that are necessitated by the various contexts. Frequently, nursing students are so conscious of their need to be professionals and use appropriate nursing language that they lose sight of the importance that changes in context make to effective interpersonal communication. While it may be necessary for a nursing student in a crisis setting to take on a more authoritative role and communication behaviors, in an emotional context, like an end-of-life setting, nurturing and supportive verbal messages will likely be much more effective. Simulations offer a real opportunity to illustrate for students the important relationship between context and communication.

As simulations are developed with a goal of assessing interpersonal communication behaviors and interpersonal relationship building, faculty can create situations to explore how students demonstrate critical skills. For example, scenarios can encourage and assess a student's ability to introduce himself or herself to patients and relatives. By having patients, relatives, peers, or team members in simulations describe and discuss various information, faculty can assess a student's ability to use active listening skills. Too often, students are so aware of what information they need to communicate and/or gather instead of focusing and listening to what the other person is saying or asking. These simulations afford faculty an opportunity to evaluate student's active listening skills, such as the following:

- Concentrating on what the other person is saying instead of the next question
- Leaning toward the speaker
- Taking occasional notes, if needed
- Providing feedback to assure understanding and demonstrate listening

The importance of feedback and how students demonstrate their listening skills is critical to the sender of a message, but using listening skills to evaluate a patient, relative, peer, or team member's communication is equally important. Simulations provide faculty the opportunity to assess both the student's ability to provide appropriate feedback as well as evaluate his or her skills at communicating feedback to the sender of a message.

These assessments are very important because communication research has shown how interpersonal communication behaviors impact relationship building (Burgoon & Hale, 1984; Gibb, 1991; Pearson, Nelson, Titsworth, & Harter, 2006). Humans are more accepting of information and recommendations from individuals they find credible and trustworthy. How nursing students demonstrate their verbal and nonverbal communication skills helps to determine how they will be assessed by patients, relatives, peers, and team members in terms of competency and credibility.

Simulations also afford faculty the opportunity to help assure that students are not using stereotyping in their communication. By developing scenarios that utilize various cultures or situations, faculty can observe and listen to the students' communication to determine if stereotyping is occurring. For example, a scenario with a homeless person could be developed to help assess whether students are using stereotyping in their verbal or nonverbal communication. The student not introducing herself or himself, calling the patient by his or her first name without asking permission, and minimizing touching the patient could all be examples of communication behaviors that demonstrate stereotyping and the need for intervention by faculty. Such simulations afford faculty the opportunity to not only evaluate student use of stereotyping but also how they respond, verbally and nonverbally, to the verbal and nonverbal behaviors of patients, relatives, peers, and/or team members.

Another key aspect of nursing communication that can be evaluated using simulations is how students handle conflict. Scenarios can be developed to assess how students respond to a variety of conflicts:

- Nurse–patient
- Nurse–family
- Peer–peer
- Nurse–team member

In addition, simulations can be developed to challenge students to use de-escalation techniques, such as with an agitated patient, to effectively manage conflict and enhance communication exchange and outcomes.

Simulations are an excellent tool for improving group communication skills. Scenarios can be designed to assess how a student interacts with a variety of team members and how the student responds, verbally and nonverbally, to a crisis situation. Also, a simulation can be created to explore how students communicate to other team members about a patient at the bedside. Or, a scenario could be developed to illustrate how a student, a dietitian, and a physician would work together to counsel relatives in a home care setting about a patient's treatment plan and prognosis.

The successful transfer of health information between nursing students and patients, relatives, peers, and/or team members requires effective intrapersonal, interpersonal, and group communication skills. Simulations afford faculty and nursing students an excellent and unique opportunity to enhance students' verbal and nonverbal communication. By creating scenarios that simultaneously challenge students' clinical and communication skills, faculty have the rare opportunity of observing and evaluating how students think, assess, react, and communicate in diverse contexts using verbal and nonverbal behaviors. Simulations provide faculty the ability to assess how students communicate verbally and nonverbally and help to assure that their nursing students will be able to effectively assess, educate, and empower patients. Simulations provide a 21st-century mechanism for improving education and assessment through direct observation of students' biopsychosocial skills in a safe, controlled environment.

Scenarios do not need to be long or complicated. Short scenarios with one key point and lasting 5 minutes may be sufficient. For example, students in their first clinical course or in a new clinical area find it difficult to anticipate the types of questions they may be asked by patients and family. One approach is to craft a scenario where the student walks into the patient's room, makes an introduction, and is asked a question by the patient. The scenario can be stopped at this point, and the faculty member can ask all the students how they might appropriately respond to this patient's question. After obtaining responses and discussing various options, students can test which response might be the best by allowing the scenario to continue. Once the communication is ended, the scenario can end. The debriefing time can be spent discussing the success or failure of the communicated information to adequately address the patient's question as well as other possible approaches to the situation.

To aid in the development of simulations that also include an opportunity for faculty to observe, challenge, and evaluate student health communication skills, please refer to the checklist that follows.

Health Communication in Scenarios Checklist

Note: Not all elements listed below may be necessary or appropriate for all scenarios.

- ☐ Has the scenario been developed to evaluate the student's ability to determine the biological, sociological, and psychological aspects of the patient's or family member's illness, injury, or situation?
- ☐ Does the scenario provide an opportunity to assess how the student uses intrapersonal communication to assess the situation and communication (can the student's thinking be evaluated by the verbal and nonverbal behaviors required in the scenario)?
- ☐ Are there behaviors in the scenario designed to assess the student's nonverbal communication with patient, peers, other providers, and/or family members?

☐ Has the scenario been developed in a way that will help the student demonstrate his or her effective use of appropriate health literacy based on the patient or family member included in the interaction?

☐ Will the scenario provide a mechanism to assess the student's active listening and/or empathic listening skills and behaviors?

☐ Are cameras positioned to capture nonverbal communications and active listening behaviors of the student?

☐ Does the scenario guidance include directions for the students to specifically observe for communication patterns?

☐ Have questions been developed for the debriefing process that specifically address the various forms of communications that are the focus of the scenario?

☐ Does the scenario encourage the student to practice his or her interpersonal relationship-building and interpersonal communication skills?

    ☐ Appropriate introduction/greeting

    ☐ Eye contact

    ☐ Smiling or appropriate facial expressions

    ☐ Handshake

    ☐ Appropriate use of space/kinesics

    ☐ Appropriate use of haptics/touch

    ☐ Minimal interruptions of the patient, family member, and/or peer

    ☐ Seeking feedback to assure effective communication

    ☐ Providing feedback to illustrate listening competencies and minimize miscommunication

    ☐ Requesting permission from the patient before touching for examination or attaching equipment (blood pressure cuff, pulse oximeter analyzer, etc.)

    ☐ Using appropriate tone, volume, and pitch for the setting (e.g., nonemergent vs. emergency)

☐ Does the scenario provide an opportunity to assess any stereotyping the student might be using in his or her communication with the patient or family member?

☐ Will the scenario assess the student's ability to appropriately close conversations (not asking questions while leaving the room or seeking feedback with a hand on the door knob, etc.)?

☐ Was the scenario developed in a way that allows an instructor to assess the student's ability to educate the patient and/or family about any number of topics related to the situation (biological, sociological, or psychological)?

References

Arford, P. (2005). Nurse-physician communication: An organizational accountability. *Nurse Economic$, 23*(2), 72–77.

Aspden, P., Wolcott, J. A., Bootman, J. L., & Cronenwett, R. L. (Eds.). (2008). *Preventing medication errors.* Washington, DC: The National Academies Press.

Birdwhistell, R. (1970). *Kinesics and context.* Philadelphia: University of Pennsylvania Press.

Burgoon, J., & Hale, J. (1984). The fundamental topoi of relational communication. *Communication Monographs, 51,* 193–214.

Gibb, J. (1991). *Trust: A new vision of human relationships for business, education, family, and personal living* (2nd ed.). North Hollywood, CA: Newcastle Publishing.

Hall, E. (1959). *The silent language*. New York: Doubleday.

Leonard, M., Graham, S., & Bonacum, D. (2004). The human factor: The critical importance of effective teamwork and communication in providing safe care. *Quality & Safety Health Care, 13*(Suppl. 1), i85–i90.

Lyman, S., & Scott, M. (1967). Territoriality: A neglected social dimension. *Social Problems, 15*, 235–249.

Mayo, E. (1945). *The social problems of an industrialized civilization*. Boston: Harvard University.

Mehrabian, A. (1981). *Silent messages: Implicit communication of emotion and attitudes* (2nd ed.). Belmont, CA: Wadsworth.

Pearson, J., Nelson, P., Titsworth, S., & Harter, L. (2006). *Human communication* (2nd ed.). Boston: McGraw-Hill.

Rosenfeld, L., & Civikly, J. (1976). *With words unspoken: The nonverbal experience*. New York: Holt, Rinehart & Winston.

Shockley-Zalabak, P. (2006). *Fundamentals of organizational communication: Knowledge, sensitivity, skills, values* (6th ed.) Boston: Allyn and Bacon.

Trenholm, S., & Jensen, A. (2008). *Interpersonal communication* (6th ed.). New York: Oxford University Press.

Washington University School of Medicine. (2006, December 26). Clinical simulation technology used to improve communication of medical teams. *Science Daily*. Retrieved February 11, 2008, from http://www.sciencedaily.com/releases/2006/12/061222092321.htm

WHO Collaborating Centres for Patient Safety Solutions. (2007). Communication during patient hand-overs. *Patient Safety Solutions, 1*, Solution 3.

Wood, J. (2005). *Gendered lives: Communication, gender, & culture* (6th ed.). Belmont, CA: Thomson-Wadsworth.

Innovative Simulation Scenarios in Diverse Settings

In keeping with the purpose of this book, Part II presents the scenarios created by contributors invited to discuss the implementation of simulation-based pedagogy in each contributor's individualized teaching. A wide variety of scenarios were selected to showcase the flexibility of using simulation throughout the nursing curriculum. While the majority of scenarios available in nursing education are medical-surgical, the following scenarios show the wide range use of simulation in all areas of nursing, including mental health, pediatrics, and obstetrics. While most are created by the primary instructor in the courses they lead, we have also included senior competency scenarios, student-generated scenarios, and an example of collaborative scenarios between nursing students and medical residents.

Each chapter follows templates created by the editors. These chapter and scenario templates represent a synthesis of the editors' combined expertise in scenario generation and presentation. In the gathering and editing of the following chapters, we have refined the presentation of the chapter and scenarios into what the editors feel represent the best practices in scenario generation.

In the chapter template, each contributor tells his or her own story on the integration and use of simulation in teaching and describes the educational institutions simulation facilities. Objectives for the simulation are outlined, and an introduction to the scenario is described, including setting the scene, technology used, objectives, and a description of the participants. Contributors also detail the running of the scenario, present the completed scenario template, and offer debriefing guidelines and suggestions and key features for further use. We also asked each contributor to give recommendations for further use and discuss how simulation-based pedagogy has contributed to improved student outcomes.

The scenario template was designed to be lifted from the chapter as "ready-to-use" scenarios. These templates include the title, focus area, and a scenario description. Scenario objectives are included along with the American Association of Colleges of Nursing (AACN), National Council of State Boards of Nursing (NCSBN), and National League for Nursing (NLN) focus areas addressed in the scenario. A detailed description of how to set up the scenario, equipment and resources required, and the recommended level of fidelity of the human patient simulator are also described by each contributor. The scenario implementation is included, and evaluative criteria are outlined.

Although the chapter and scenario templates have been standardized throughout this part, the editors believe that scenarios should be as flexible and creative as the educators who use them. Those new to simulation in nursing education ask "Where do I begin" or "How can I get started?" We have all been overwhelmed by what seems a daunting task of implementing simulation-based pedagogy. There is no prescribed idea, and there are many stories and perspectives presented in this part. It is the hope of the editors that these scenario chapters will inspire and energize enthusiastic educators to make simulation "real" in their own nursing education curriculum.

Scenario Chapter Template

A. Discussion of implementation of simulation-based pedagogy in each contributor's individualized teaching
B. Description of educational materials available in your teaching area and relative to your specialty
C. Specific objective for simulation utilization within a specific course and the overall program
D. Introduction of scenario to include setting the scene, technology used, objectives, and description of participants
E. Describe running of the scenario
F. Presentation of completed template (see Scenario Template below)
G. Debriefing guidelines
H. Suggestions/Key features to replicate or improve
I. Recommendations for further use
J. Discussion of simulation-based pedagogy and how this new technology has contributed to improved student outcomes

Scenario Template

The scenario template information is included in chapter template Section F for each chapter.

Title:
Include course description (generic), such as Pain Management, Early Medical-Surgical course; 2nd-semester junior-year BSN or 1st-semester freshman-year ADN

Focus Area:
Medical-Surgical, Obstetrics, Pediatrics, Intensive Care Units, Senior Scenario

Scenario Description:
Include patient demographics (gender, age, race, religion, occupation, height and weight), pertinent past medical history, presenting symptoms, illnesses, injuries and recent surgeries, current medications, allergies, significant others, social history, mental health history.

Scenario Objectives:
AACN/NCSBN/NLN focus area(s) addressed (e.g., from AACN)
http://www.aacn.nche.edu/Education/pdf/BEdraft.pdf

Setting the Scene:
Equipment needed: Simulator, video recording device, medical equipment (e.g., patient monitor, oxygen hook-up, bandages, pulse oximeter, blood pressure cuff, stethoscope), medical record (electronic or paper)

Resources needed: Textbooks, computer access for database search and evidence-based practice, personal digital assistant for point-of-care decision making—specifically, student and faculty instructions for preparation (any psychomotor skills or cognitive activities that would enhance student preparation)

Simulator level: High fidelity, moderate fidelity, static manikin, live patients, video clips—think outside the box!

Participants needed: Number, roles identified, and scripts (if needed)

Scenario Implementation:

Initial settings for human patient simulator
Required student assessments and actions—checklist of actions accomplished, objectives met, assessments demonstrated
Instructor interventions—how the instructor might facilitate student success, any anticipated "out-of-protocol" occurrences, how students are present to learn, how many students, and may students choose to take another turn? Can they practice until they master it?

Evaluative Criteria:

Refer back to clearly defined learning objectives
Determine how to evaluate if criteria have been met (develop a rubric for exceeded expectations, met objectives, below expectations)

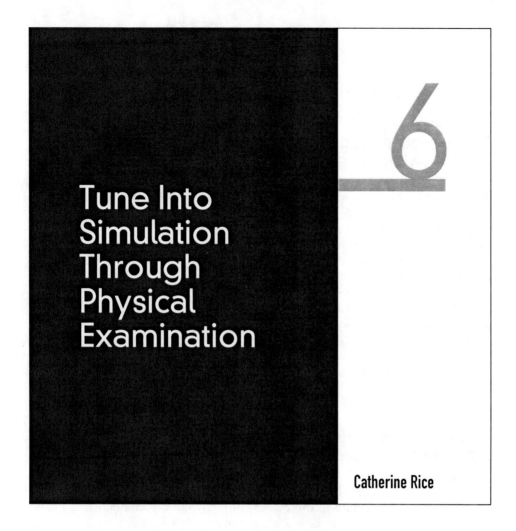

Tune Into Simulation Through Physical Examination

6

Catherine Rice

A. Discussion of Implementation of Simulation-Based Pedagogy in Each Contributor's Individualized Teaching

As a teacher of physical assessment skills, I have had the opportunity to educate my students regarding how essential it is for them to learn, develop, and eventually master the skills of inspection, palpation, percussion, and auscultation. I try to instill in them a vivid awareness of the need to create an assessment environment that will allow the nurse to maximize the accuracy of this assessment process while also instilling patient confidence in that process. As such, I emphasize the need to ensure that each student follows a structured, well-organized, and comprehensive preparation and execution process prior to and during each assessment activity. I note to my students that this requirement is just as important when they use simulation technology as when dealing with real patients in order to establish a routine they will consistently use to ensure that each step of this process is consistently followed. The use of simulation technology is especially useful in creating the equivalent of "muscle memory" for the students because of the ability to do frequent and repetitive exercises using this technology. It is especially useful in assisting students to learn, develop, and mature their assessment skills.

B. Description of Educational Materials Available in Your Teaching Area and Relative to Your Specialty

The Nursing Department program offerings include a BS, RN to BS, and MS degree. The university houses three separate nursing laboratories, each tailored for specific patient environments. These include an acute care, chronic care, and subacute care setting. Each of the simulation rooms is equipped with scenario-appropriate equipment. Items such as hospital beds, stretchers, fluid infusion devices, fluid drainage systems, monitoring systems, high-fidelity human patient simulators (HPS), crash carts, ventilators, and bedside tables are available for creating a tailored scenario. Props such as clothing, eyeglasses, dentures, wigs, splints, wounds, compression boots, and miscellaneous other items are readily available to allow the instructor to create a wide range of different patient dispositions. A video recording device is available to capture student performance and is subsequently used to debrief students regarding their performance.

C. Specific Objectives for Simulation Utilization Within a Specific Course and the Overall Program

The overall objective of this simulation scenario is to define parameters of physical assessment for faculty in the context of simulation technology and create an awareness of the need to develop and nurture these skills through the use of simulation technology. Traditionally, physical assessment has been taught in the classroom through a variety of techniques, including lectures, videos, faculty demonstrations, student partnering, and such, and generally concluding in students demonstrating accurate assessment skills on completion of each module. In an era of evolving technology, nursing graduates must be introduced to and equipped to manage the complexities of the technologic environment they will encounter. During each physical assessment module, simulation technology can be a valuable educational tool for both faculty and students. While we may rely on technology to provide health care personnel with useful patient information (such as heart rhythm using an EKG reading), it is important for students to recognize that although the EKG looks perfect in rhythm, rate, form, and amplitude, the patient could be dead. Students are taught that a diagnosis of "pulseless electrical activity," or PEA, means that the patient is clinically dead. Electrical conductivity of the heart, although present on a monitoring device, does not necessarily mean the patient is alive. Therefore, it must be stressed to students that technology, although useful, is limited and is only one of many tools that should be accessed from their assessment tool kit. In fact, it is essential that students first develop and mature their personal assessment skills of inspection, palpation, percussion, and auscultation and then use technology to validate and refine the effectiveness of those skills.

To teach the art of assessment skills (*inspection, palpation, percussion,* and *auscultation*), faculty can direct students to think of themselves as "instruments" to be "tuned" into the process of assessment techniques. As musicians learn to tune their instruments, so too must student nurses learn to tune into physical assessment.

A second objective of this simulation scenario is to provide a generic teaching template for each physical assessment module that can be tailored by the individual faculty member and includes structured, supportive, and evaluative elements. Learning modules are developed to be prescriptive in nature and are designed with the intent that the student will master simple components of the assessment process in a step-by-step sequence before progressing to more complex assessment techniques. Students who successfully complete individual learning modules advance, while those who are unsuccessful are offered additional learning opportunities or experiences and remediation activities within an agreeable time frame. Prior to initiation of the module, students are provided with an evaluative/assessment rubric. On mastery of the module, the student may receive a "satisfactory" or "pass" as a part of a credentialing process. If the student is unsuccessful and unable to perform the assessment, the instructor advises the student in the following manner:

1. Have student self-evaluate performance using the corresponding skill performance checklist
2. Instructor provides feedback on student evaluation to identify areas of strength and areas requiring improvement
3. Instructor and student develop an individualized remedial plan, to include the following:
   a. A review of specific scenario requirements and expectations
   b. Student practicing specific skills in a nonrisk environment
   c. Student re-performs the required assessment skills for validation by instructor

The timing of each module must be carefully planned and flows from the course content. In addition, the student who attends to the readings and corresponding available media (video demonstrations, etc.) tends to move quickly and efficiently through the learning process. Students should be counseled, however, as to the necessity to review and reflect on their performance regardless of how rapidly they appear to be progressing. A formalized reflection process creates an opportunity for students to identify and articulate positive behaviors, areas for improvement, and methods to enhance or address these areas. Weekly reflections, however brief, serve to demonstrate to the student his or her unique development and provide positive reinforcement of the progress being made. Having students identify what they do that contributes to improving their own performance and then having these students share, anonymously, this information with their fellow students can foster a positive communal learning experience.

D. Introduction of Scenario to Include Setting the Scene, Technology Used, Objectives, and Description of Participants

Setting the Scene and Technology Used

The scene takes place in a long-term care nursing facility. The patient, an 84-year-old female, is complaining of right leg pain and feeling dizzy. The student nurse is assigned to conduct a general health assessment followed by a physical examination. On completion of the assessments, the student nurse will prioritize an individualized plan of care.

The patient will be a high-fidelity HPS. She will be dressed in her nightgown, lying on her hospital bed, covered to her chest with a sheet, and in a semiprivate room with a female roommate of similar age in an accompanying bed. There will be a wheelchair next to her bed, and overbed table, a telephone, a call bell, and a water pitcher with a plastic cup. The patient's head of bed is elevated 15 degrees, only one side rail is raised, the bed is in the lowest position with locks secured, and the patient is sleeping on student arrival. The privacy curtain between the beds is open and the lights are dimmed. The person operating the simulator will be allowed to answer questions and speak for the patient.

The student will be provided with an opportunity to obtain all necessary equipment and forms prior to entering the patient's room. Equipment needed include the following: simulator, video recording device, assessment tools such as alcohol hand sanitizer, clean gloves, blood pressure cuff, stethoscope, medical record, and so forth.

Objectives

1. Conduct a general survey of a patient.
2. Obtain a health history and complete a physical examination.

Description of Participants

1. *Student nurse in long-term care rotation:* The student should be prepared in patient assessment techniques, including *inspection, palpation, percussion,* and *auscultation.* The student should be knowledgeable about the equipment and forms necessary to accomplish this task. The student should obtain the necessary tools and forms from the instructor prior to entering the patient's room.
2. *An 84-year-old female patient in a long-term care setting:* This role will be played by a high-fidelity HPS. The HPS will be lying down on her bed. The simulator operator will respond with short, simple answers to questions posed by the student and will indicate that she does not understand when questions are not presented in clear, simple terms. The "patient" should not volunteer any information and should indicate a degree of self-consciousness and hesitancy when "personal" questions are asked.
3. *Instructor running the scenario:* The person running the scenario will also be operating the HPS (a high-fidelity simulator), unless another qualified

operator is available. In that case, the instructor running the scenario will observe and take notes relative to scenario objectives.

E. Describe Running of the Scenario

The student will be given guidance as to the specific objectives of the assignment. The student will be told the time of day the assessment will be occurring and will be provided with a basic health history of the patient based on forms the patient had completed when she first expressed concerns regarding a change in her health status. The student will be expected to identify the tools and forms needed to conduct the assessment and will be given those tools and forms requested. After making an introduction and explaining the purpose of the visit, the student should request permission of the patient to begin the interview assessment.

F. Presentation of Completed Template

Title: General Health Assessment and Physical Examination

Focus Area:
Assessment techniques include inspection, palpation, percussion, and auscultation.

Scenario Description:
This chapter introduces concepts and techniques of physical assessment in the context of the nursing process. Simulation experiences provide opportunities to develop assessment skills in preparation for clinical courses in a minimal-risk environment. In addition, the simulation can be repeated as often as necessary for the student to gain confidence without exposing actual patients to the student's learning process.

Prescenario setup checklist: Equip your examination area with the following (Jarvis, 2008):

Examination table
Simulation device (man, woman, or child)
Privacy screening
Wall-mounted or gooseneck stand lamp
Rolling stool
Bedside stand or table
Documentation (pen or pencil and forms)

Equipment:

Platform scale with height attachment
Skinfold calipers
Sphygmomanometer
Stethoscope with bell and diaphragm end pieces

Thermometer
Pulse oximeter
Flashlight or penlight
Otoscope/ophthalmoscope
Tuning fork
Nasal speculum
Tongue depressor
Pocket vision screener
Skin-marking pen
Flexible tape measure and ruler marked in centimeters
Reflex hammer
Sharp object (split tongue blade)
Cotton balls
Clean gloves
Fecal occult blood test materials
Gastric pH test strips (pp. 137–138)

On a note card: Provide the following information about the patient to the student: patient's name, demographics (gender, age, race, religion, occupation, height and weight), pertinent past medical history, presenting symptoms, illnesses, injuries and recent surgeries, current medications, allergies, significant other factors, social history, mental health history, and any other pertinent information. Identify your patient by name (first and last). Note style of the following Patient Data Form.

Patient Data Form:

Name:

Demographics:

Pertinent Past Medical History:

Presenting Symptoms, Illnesses, Injuries and Recent Surgeries:

Current Medications:

Allergies:

Significant Other Factors:

Social History:

Mental Health History:

Scenario alternatives: If a high-fidelity HPS is unavailable, alternative simulation approaches would be to utilize a medium-fidelity simulator with student volunteers or other faculty to role-play.

Evaluative Criteria:

Required Student Assessment and Actions

1. _____ *Hand hygiene:* Demonstrate performance of correct hand hygiene.
2. _____ *Equipment:* Gather the appropriate equipment, and check that the equipment is functional prior to entering the examination area.

3. _____ *Documentation:* Gather documentation paperwork prior to entering the examination area, and validate that it is appropriate for this specific procedure.

4. _____ *Request entry:* Knock on patient's door to request entry to examination area.

5. _____ *Personal introduction:* Introduce yourself (student identification (ID) badge must be visible, but do not rely on your name tag to serve as your introduction).

6. _____ *Confirm patient identity:* Identify patient (ID band or whatever is deemed appropriate). If your patient does not have identification, then the student should not proceed until the patient's identity is verified and an appropriate ID band is placed on the patient.

7. _____ *State purpose:* "I'd like your permission and cooperation to perform the following examination. . . ."

8. _____ *Query patient concerns:* Ask whether the patient has any questions, concerns, or other issues prior to start of the exam. It is important for students to recognize that in order to have a successful experience with the patient, the patient's immediate needs must be met prior to the initiation of an examination.

9. _____ *Visually survey the patient:* During this introductory phase, it is important to visually survey the patient as well as his or her environment.
   a. _____ Note whether the patient is awake, alert, and responsive or not.
   b. _____ Note patient's disposition (e.g., lying, sitting, standing, etc.)
   c. _____ Note the condition of the patient's physical environment (temperature of the room, cleanliness, equipment in use or on standby).
   d. _____ Note tubes, drains, IVs, etc.; identify what is present and, if there is a drainage amount, note its color, the presence of odor, etc. (For each scenario, the faculty can manipulate the simulation environment to create a realistic patient disposition and setting.)

10. _____ *Set up examination field:* Have the student decide where to set up the examination field, assessing for cleanliness, clutter, garbage, etc. (The student may need to clean off the patient's overbed tray table, wipe down the surface to assure cleanliness, etc.)

11. _____ Have the student practice/demonstrate physical examination assessment module, providing corrective feedback as appropriate.

Scenario concluding steps: On completion of the documentation of the physical examination module, the student is expected to do the following:

1. Provide an opportunity for patient to express concerns, questions, or seek clarification.
2. Thank patient for his or her participation and cooperation.
3. Document according to physical examination guidelines.
4. Place patient's bed height in the lowest position (if raised during the examination).
5. Lock wheels of bed, and reset safety alarms/devices as appropriate.
6. Assure that patient's personal dignity is maintained.
7. Assure that patient's call system is within easy access, and ask patient to demonstrate how he or she would call for help/assistance if needed using the call system.

8. Position patient's assistive devices, bedside tray, and water pitcher, etc., within patient's reach.
9. Discuss with patient what happens next (what should he or she expect, what is expected of him or her, who to turn to for assistance).
10. Determine who has permission for status updates.

G. Debriefing Guidelines

Instructor may debrief students individually or as a group.

1. Review learning objectives.
2. Students verbally recap the events as they remember them chronologically.
3. Students will identify specific areas for improvement and end with their positive behaviors/critical thinking.
4. Students will complete a written reflection exercise within 24 to 48 hours.
5. Faculty posts insightful student reflections anonymously for communal enrichment with student permission.
6. Instructor provides personalized feedback to students.

H. Suggestions/Key Features to Replicate or Improve

The advantages of using high-fidelity HPS are multifaceted and include the ability for frequent repetition of exercises, real time, and realistic feedback as well as an ability to avoid harm to the patients during our student nurse learning continuum. The use of high-fidelity HPS can be enhanced by creating a variety of scenarios across a wide spectrum of patient care settings.

The technology must be monitored regularly for optimum functioning. Suggestions for maintenance and updates are as follows:

1. Identify appropriate resource personnel responsible for the maintenance and updates of the simulation technology.
2. Identify service schedule for all simulation equipment and mechanism for reporting issues.
3. Identify users, and establish training program.

I. Recommendations for Further Use

Tuning into physical assessment through the use of simulation technology is a wonderful teaching tool. Faculty should remember that "keeping it simple" is not always so simple or easily mastered by the student nurse. In order for the student to develop competency in basic assessment skills, patience, time, and practice are necessary. In addition, the use of positive feedback is critical for creating a successful learning experience.

J. Discussion of Simulation-Based Pedagogy and How This New Technology Has Contributed to Improved Student Outcomes

Students utilize an end-of-semester course evaluation to provide faculty with feedback regarding the use of high-fidelity HPS technology in the laboratory setting. While students report a very positive learning experience directly on completion of the course, the more compelling argument that this use of technology has merit is based on their actual encounters with patients in subsequent clinical visits. The competency level of students noted while they are engaged in the physical assessment of their patients is overwhelming evidence that basic physical assessment skills developed through simulation are transferable to the patient setting.

Reference

Jarvis, C. (2008). *Physical examination and health assessment* (5th ed.). St. Louis: MO: Saunders Elsevier Inc.

Recommended Texts

Potter, P., & Perry, A. (2005). *Fundamentals of nursing* (6th ed.). St. Louis: MO: Mosby Elsevier Inc.

Smeltzer, S. C., & Bare, B. (2006). *Brunner and Suddarth's textbook of medical-surgical nursing* (11th ed.). Philadelphia: Lippincott Williams & Wilkins.

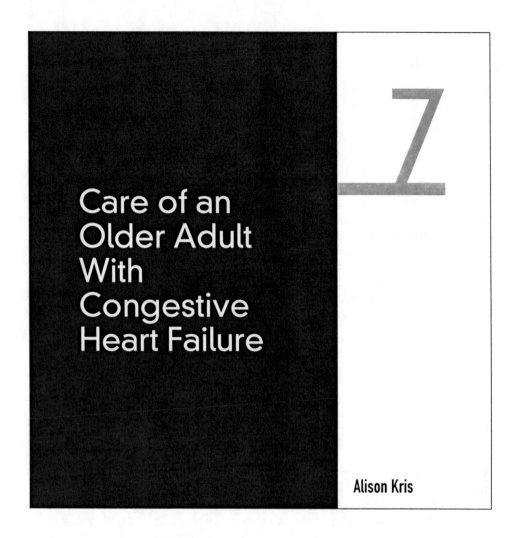

7

Care of an Older Adult With Congestive Heart Failure

Alison Kris

A. Discussion of Implementation of Simulation-Based Pedagogy in Each Contributor's Individualized Teaching

As the geriatrics content is typically offered at the sophomore level, elementary simulations allow faculty to introduce foundational content essential to the care of older adults. Examples of content reinforced through the use of scenarios has included (1) differentiating delirium, dementia, and depression and (2) distinguishing normal from abnormal changes of aging.

Individual faculty at Fairfield University have also had the opportunity to participate in a faculty learning community (see chapter 4). This process facilitated discussions about the goals and expected outcomes associated with the use of simulations. In addition, there was discussion of the pedagogical theory supporting the use of simulations to enhance the delivery of nursing content.

B. Description of Educational Materials Available in Your Teaching Area and Relative to Your Specialty

The Fairfield University School of Nursing's Robin Kanarek Learning Resource Center is a state-of-the-art facility that provides nursing students with the opportunity to participate in realistic patient care scenarios. The Center is comprised of a simulation room, a control room, and an adjacent classroom enabling classes of up to 35 students to view the ongoing scenario as it progresses. A high-fidelity human patient simulator (HPS) allows students to assess the typical vital signs and lung sounds of a nursing home resident with an acute exacerbation of congestive heart failure (CHF). In addition, through a partnership with the Emergisoft Corporation, the center houses realistic computer interfaces similar to what students will find in the clinical practice arena, including electronic medical records. In the following scenario, students will use an actual computer interface to access patient lab values and history.

C. Specific Objective for Simulation Utilization Within a Specific Course and the Overall Program

This scenario is intended for students enrolled in Geriatric Nursing, a sophomore-level course in a 4-year baccalaureate nursing program. The course focuses on the nursing care of older adults living in long-term care settings. Building on skills developed in a previous course in health assessment, normal physiological changes of aging and related assessment skills are incorporated into this course. Management of common geriatric care problems is emphasized. As the first clinical course in the nursing curriculum, students will also be provided with the opportunity to develop an understanding of how the nursing role merges with life goals, philosophy, and meaning and to use those values to develop professional behaviors consistent with these aspects of life.

D. Introduction of Scenario to Include Setting the Scene, Technology Used, Objectives, and Description of Participants

Setting the Scene

The simulation will take place in a nursing home. The resident will be in bed, in his or her room. A certified nursing assistant (CNA) will provide a report on the resident.

Technology Used

This simulation will make use of a medium- or high-fidelity HPS with the capacity to transmit respiratory sounds, a video recording device, simulated oxygen, pulse oximeter, blood pressure cuff, stethoscope, electronic medical record, water pitcher, call light, and ID bracelet. The patient should be wearing a diaper.

Objectives

Nursing students will be required to evaluate and manage the complex and dynamic hydration status of the older adult nursing home patient suffering from CHF. This simulation will include evaluating the nursing home resident for signs and symptoms of both dehydration and overhydration. The scenario will test decision-making skills regarding the administration of diuretic medications and the evaluation of key laboratory values and will require communication with other nurses, physicians, and patient family members.

Description of Participants

One or two students, an instructor to act as the voice of Mrs. Fertal, a "CNA" to deliver the patient report, and a "physician" to whom students may report change of condition

E. Describe Running of the Scenario

Initial settings for the HPS:

> BP: 130/85, P: 75, RR: 17, T: 97.5
> Oxygen saturation settings should be set to 90%.
> Place note cards on the legs of the manikin indicating that she has +1 pitting edema to her ankles.
> Lung sounds with slight crackles bilaterally.
> Atrial fibrillation.
> Resident is sitting in bed in a high Fowler position.
> Place a reddened area on the patient's coccyx indicating a stage 1 pressure ulcer (use a model when available/appropriate).

F. Presentation of Completed Template

Title: Care of Older Adult With Congestive Heart Failure
This simulation is used within a geriatric course given during the second-semester sophomore year of a baccalaureate program or first-semester freshman year of an associate degree program.

Focus Area:
This scenario is geared toward sophomore-level geriatric nursing students practicing in long-term care settings.

Scenario Description:
One or two students will receive report from a CNA on nights, and some key data will be missed and/or misinterpreted (e.g., weight gain). An instructor will act as the voice of Mrs. Fertal, and a physician will be available (either by phone in the control room or physically present) for students to report changes of condition.

Nursing students will be required to evaluate and manage the complex and dynamic hydration status of the older adult nursing home patient, including evaluating the patient for signs and symptoms of both dehydration and overhydration in light of the diagnosis of CHF. The scenario will test decision-making skills regarding the administration of diuretic medications and the evaluation of key laboratory values and will require communication with other nurses, physicians, and patient family members.

Scenario Objectives:

1. Introduce self.
2. Check ID band.
3. Check vital signs, including pulse oximeter.
   - Note low pulse oximeter.
   - Note that decreased temperature is a common and normal finding in the older adult.
4. Conduct a head-to-toe assessment.
   - Note rales in bilateral bases.
   - Note pedal edema.
   - Note reddened area on coccyx.
   - Note atrial fibrillation.
5. Check the compressor to ensure that it is working and delivering the correct amount of oxygen to the patient.
6. Assess mental status for signs of acute confusion and signs of depression.
7. Student documents relevant findings: color, position, breath sounds, heart sounds, vital signs, weight, change in activity level, presence of a stage 1 pressure ulcer. While charting, student checks back to compare the current weight with the previous weight. Student checks the chart for relevant lab values.
8. Student notes that abnormal labs indicate hypovolemia: decreased blood urea nitrogen (BUN), decreased hematocrit.
9. Student contacts the physician and reports relevant findings in a cohesive way. This may be done via phone in the simulation room, which connects him or her to faculty in the control room acting as the nurse practitioner and physician.

For all scenarios, the following criteria from the American Association of Colleges of Nursing (1998) *Essentials of Baccalaureate Education for Professional Nursing Practice* were addressed:

- Employ a range of technologies that facilitate patient care, including patient education and patient safety.
- Integrate clinical data from all relevant sources of technology to inform the delivery of care.
- Use professional communication and collaborative skills to deliver evidence-based, patient-centered care.
- Conduct a basic health history, including recognition of genetic risks and environmental exposure to identify current and future health problems.
- Demonstrate the application of psychomotor skills for the efficient, safe, and compassionate delivery of patient care.

▨ Deliver appropriate patient-centered teaching that reflects developmental stage, age, culture, and health literacy considerations.
▨ Implement holistic, patient-centered care that reflects an understanding of pathophysiology, pharmacology, medical management, and nursing management across the health-illness continuum (i.e., from primary care to home care to acute care to follow-up).
▨ Implement evidence-based nursing interventions as appropriate for managing the acute and chronic care of patients and promoting health across the life span (e.g., acute and chronic pain, mobility, nutrition, skin care, oral, hydration, elimination, falls prevention, infection prevention, etc.).
▨ Recognize and manage common geriatric syndromes, described as multifactorial functional problems affecting older adults that defy simple categorization into discrete disease states.

The scenario also allows students to practice key elements from the National Council Licensure Examination for a Registered Nurse (NCLEX-RN) test plan (NCSBN, 2007) including:

Physiological Integrity

> *Basic Care and Comfort*
>   Nutrition and Oral Hydration
>   Rest and Sleep
> *Pharmacological and Parenteral Therapies*
>   Expected effects/Outcomes
>   Pharmacological Agents/Actions
> *Reduction of Risk Potential*
>   Laboratory Values
>   System Specific Assessments
>   Vital Signs
> *Physiological Adaptation*
>   Hemodynamics
>   Fluid and Electrolyte Imbalances
>   Pathophysiology

Setting the Scene:

> *Patient:* Mrs. Irma Fertal
> *Age:* 89 years
> *Allergies:* Penicillin (PCN), codeine
> *Weight:* 177.2 lb
> *Physician:* Dr. Newman
> *Major diagnoses:* CHF, chronic obstructive pulmonary disease (COPD), diabetes, hypothyroidism, atrial fibrillation, osteoarthritis of the left hip
> *Medications and orders:*
> Fluticasone propionate (Advair discus) 250/50
> Levothyroxine (Synthroid), 50 mg by mouth daily
> Predisone (Deltasone), 10 mg by mouth daily
> Wafarin (Coumadin), 5 mg by mouth daily

NPH insulin, 25 U each morning and each evening

Codeine, 2 tabs every 4 hours as needed

Oxygen, 2 L continuous

Oxygen saturation reading each evening

Lab values: Instructor may place in electronic medical record, or in HPS, a lab value sheet indicating all labs within normal range with the exception of decreased BUN and decreased hematocrit.

Scenario Part One

Setting the Scene and Patient History

Mrs. Fertal is an 89-year-old resident of White Oak Nursing Home, where she has been a resident for 5 years. She is a heavyset woman with a round pleasant face. Her white hair has grown a bit longer than it should be kept. Her nightstand and overbed tables are cluttered with all sorts of items: the TV remote, tissues, a cordless phone, used cups, packets of artificial sweetener, and a basket of other assorted necessities. She has a walker that sits in the corner of the room and a bedside commode next to the TV. On the wall at the foot of the bed, there is a bulletin board that has some photos of her family.

Recently, she has experienced increasing shortness of breath. While normally able to ambulate to the bathroom with minimal assistance, she recently has had more difficulty with ambulation. She is on oxygen 2LNC, which is delivered by a compressor that also sits next to her bed.

Certified Nursing Assistant Report

The CNA reports to you that Mrs. Fertal is refusing to get out of bed today because she is too tired. The CNA reports that she was surprised to find that Mrs. Fertal had gained almost 10 pounds since her last weight check, despite the fact that she has not been eating very well. When you arrive, you find Mrs. Fertal sitting in bed.

Subjective Report From Patient

"I just don't feel much like getting out of bed today. I'm too tired."

Required Student Assessments and Actions

1. Introduce self.
2. Check ID band.
3. Check vital signs, including pulse oximeter.
   - Note low pulse oximeter.
   - Note decreased temperature is a common and normal finding in the older adult.
4. Conduct a head-to-toe assessment.
   - Note rales in bilateral bases.
   - Note pedal edema.
   - Note reddened area on coccyx.
   - Note atrial fibrillation.
5. Check the compressor to ensure that it is working and delivering the correct amount of oxygen to the patient.
6. Assess mental status for signs of acute confusion and signs of depression.
7. Student documents relevant findings: color, position, breath sounds, heart sounds, vital signs, weight, change in activity level, presence of a stage 1

pressure ulcer. While charting, student checks back to compare the current weight with the previous weight. Student checks the chart for relevant lab values.

8. Student notes that abnormal labs indicate hypovolemia: decreased BUN, decreased hematocrit.

9. Student contacts the physician and reports relevant findings in a cohesive way. This may be done via phone in the simulation room, which connects him or her to faculty in control room acting as nurse practitioner and physician.

At the conclusion of Part One, the physician gives the order to "monitor" the patient.

Debriefing
Discussion questions for students:

> What did the students do correctly?
> Are the students forgetting anything, or was anything done incorrectly?
> What are the students' concerns about Mrs. Fertal?
> What is the cause of the concern, and why might this be a cause of concern?
> What actions do you need to take? What are the priorities?
> What is Mrs. Fertal experiencing?
> Why might she have developed a pressure ulcer?

Scenario Part Two

Setting the Scene
Mrs. Fertal is once again sitting in bed in a high Fowler position.

Certified Nursing Assistant Report
The CNA reports to you that Mrs. Fertal has gained 32 pounds since her last weight check 1 month ago. "That is so strange," says the CNA. "She really has not been eating very well." The CNA then states, "I guess that is what happens when you get old."

Subjective Report From Patient
"My feet look like footballs. I'm so tired. I just can't seem to catch my breath."

Part Two Settings for the Human Patient Simulator

BP: 160/90, P: 85, RR: 23, T: 97.2
Bounding pulse.
Oxygen saturation settings should be set to 88%.
Place note cards on the legs of the manikin, indicating that she has +3 pitting edema to her thighs.
Lung sounds with loud crackles bilaterally.
Atrial fibrillation.
Resident is sitting in bed in a high Fowler position.
Place a reddened area on the patient's coccyx, indicating a stage 2 pressure ulcer
Simulated distended neck and peripheral veins.
Simulated blue-purple lips.

Required Student Assessments and Actions

1. Introduce self.
2. Check ID band.
3. Check vital signs, including pulse oximeter
   - Note low pulse oximeter.
   - Note increase in respiratory rate.
4. Conduct a head-to-toe assessment.
   - Note rails in bilateral bases.
   - Note pedal edema.
   - Note stage 2 pressure ulcer.
   - Note atrial fibrillation.
   - Note significant weight gain.
5. Check the compressor to ensure that it is working and delivering the correct amount of oxygen to the patient.
   - Adjust the compressor as ordered.
6. Recognize the need to humidify oxygen when delivered above 2 L per minute.
7. Assess mental status for signs of acute confusion and signs of depression.
8. Student documents relevant findings: color, position, breath sounds, heart sounds, vital signs, weight, change in activity level, presence of a stage 1 pressure ulcer. While charting, student checks back to compare the current weight with the previous weight. Student checks the chart for relevant lab values.
9. Student notes that abnormal labs indicate hypovolemia: decreased BUN, decreased hematocrit.
10. Student contacts the physician and reports relevant findings in a cohesive way.

Debriefing
Discussion questions for students:

> What did the students do correctly?
> Are the students forgetting anything, or did they do anything incorrectly?
> Why might have Mrs. Fertal's pressure ulcer worsened?
> What are your concerns about Mrs. Fertal now?
> What is the cause of the concern, and why might this be a cause of concern?
> What actions do you need to take? What are the priorities?
> What is Mrs. Fertal experiencing?
> What do you think about the comment of the CNA? How might you address this?

Scenario Part Three
You receive a call back from Dr. Newman, who gives you the following order: "Increase Lasix to 80 mg BID, increase oxygen PRN to maintain O2 sat above 92%." She has been on this new Lasix regimen for 3 days.

Setting the Scene
Mrs. Fertal is once again sitting in bed in a high Fowler position. She is wearing two diapers.

Certified Nursing Assistant Report

The CNA reports to you that Mrs. Fertal said she started feeling very dizzy when being transferred into her shower chair. She states that Mrs. Fertal is usually an "easy transfer" but that today her legs were weak and she almost fell.

Subjective Report From Patient

"I am just so dizzy . . . my head is spinning. I feel like I might pass out."

Part Three Settings for the Human Patient Simulator

BP: 90/60, P: 110, RR: 20, T: 99.2
Weight: 150 lb
Oxygen saturation settings should be set to 94%.
Legs are now without any edema.
Lung sounds are clear.
Atrial fibrillation.
Resident is sitting in bed in a high Fowler position.
Place a reddened area on the patient's coccyx indicating a stage 2 pressure ulcer.
Place two diapers on the resident.

Lab Values

All labs are within normal range with the exception of an elevated BUN, elevated BUN creatinine ratio, and a decreased potassium. Hematocrit is higher than previously noted, although still within range.

Required Student Assessments and Actions

1. Introduce self.
2. Check ID band.
3. Check vital signs, including pulse oximeter.
   - Check for orthostatic hypotension.
   - Note increased temperature as a sign of dehydration.
4. Conduct a head-to-toe assessment.
   - Note condition of mucous membranes.
5. Check the compressor to ensure that it is working and delivering the correct amount of oxygen to the patient.
6. Student documents relevant findings: color, position, breath sounds, heart sounds, vital signs, weight, change in activity level, presence of a stage 2 pressure ulcer. While charting, student checks back to compare the current weight with the previous weight and notes discrepancy. Student checks the chart for relevant lab values.
7. Student notes that abnormal labs indicate hypovolemia: increased BUN, increased BUN creatinine ratio, increased hematocrit. In addition, student notes hypokalemia.
8. Student contacts the physician and reports relevant findings in a cohesive way. The student notes the lab abnormalities and asks about holding the next dose of Lasix. The physician gives the order for .9NS at 150 mL per hour × 3 L.

G. Debriefing Guidelines

Discussion questions for students:

> What are your concerns about Mrs. Fertal?
> What is the cause of the concern, and why might this be a cause of concern?
> What actions do you need to take? What are the priorities?
> What is Mrs. Fertal experiencing?
> Why might Mrs. Fertal have two diapers on? How might you handle this, and what might you say to the CNA?
> What is missing from the physician orders? Does Mrs. Fertal need anything else?

H. Suggestions/Key Features to Replicate or Improve

Faculty may wish to review the pathophysiology of common causes of short-ness of breath in the older adult such as CHF, COPD, and pneumonia. Facilitate discussion among students about how these diseases may present differently from each other as well as how they may present in atypical ways in the older adult.

Faculty may also wish to review Starling's law, the concepts of cardiac preload and afterload, and how each of these concepts apply in this particular case. A discussion about the issues related to the use of Furosemide (Lasix) in the older adult may naturally follow.

I. Recommendations for Further Use

There are several different ways this scenario can be modified depending on the content area and audience. A unit on communication may have the student contact a worried daughter and communicate the resident's change in health or may center on how to improve communication between CNAs and other nursing staff. A student in a clinical nurse leader track may wish to explore the multiple quality of care issues (such as the development of a pressure ulcer) that arise in this case and devise ways to improve the process of care.

J. Discussion of Simulation-Based Pedagogy and How This New Technology Has Contributed to Improved Student Outcomes

Because this simulation is carried out in front of the class, students may be more motivated to arrive to class prepared. This method can also help students make the sometimes difficult leap of translating the theory they read in their textbooks into clinical practice. Instructors may tailor simulations to mimic those situations students are likely to encounter on their clinical units in order to enhance clinical performance.

References

American Association of Colleges of Nursing. (1998). *Essentials of baccalaureate education for professional nursing practice*. Washington, DC: AACN.

National Council of State Boards of Nursing. (2007). *NCLEX-RN examination: Test plan for the National Council Licensure Examination for Registered Nurses*. Retrieved June 18, 2008, from https://www.ncsbn.org/RN_Test_Plan_2007_Web.pdf

Additional Resources

Signs and symptoms of hypervolemia and hypovolemia in the geriatric client adapted from The Hartford Institute for Geriatric Nursing, *ConsultGeriRN.org*, http://www.consultgerirn.org/topics/normal_aging_changes/want_to_know_more

Discussion questions adapted from The Carnegie Foundation, *Integrative teaching at its best: Study of nursing education*, 2007. Retrieved February 27, 2008, from http://www.carnegiefoundation.org/programs/sub.asp?key=1829&subkey=2309&topkey=1829

Acknowledgment

This case was developed from data gathered from a research grant provided by the John A. Hartford Foundation.

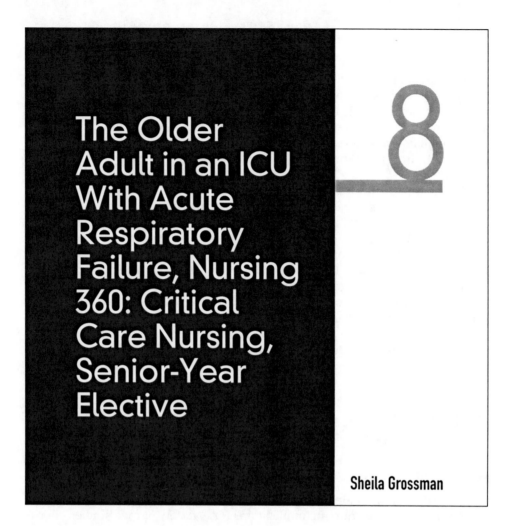

The Older Adult in an ICU With Acute Respiratory Failure, Nursing 360: Critical Care Nursing, Senior-Year Elective

8

Sheila Grossman

A & B. Discussion of Implementation of Simulation-Based Pedagogy in Contributor's Individualized Teaching and Description of Educational Materials Available in Your Institution Relative to Your Specialty

As a faculty member committed to doing interactive teaching/learning, I have worked in simulation laboratories as a critical care instructor at two large teaching medical centers and have also taught undergraduate senior nursing students for multiple years. Currently, I am involved in using a high-fidelity human patient simulator (HPS) and role-play as well as running the scenario "on the fly" with our Learning Resource director and project director for a complex scenario, "The Older Adult in an ICU with Acute Respiratory Failure," using MicroSim in Critical Care classes and setting up clinical situations. Some of the clinical situations outlined in classes include mock code, troubleshooting chronic ambulatory peritoneal dialysis (CAPD), managing pulmonary artery catheter, central venous pressure (CVP) monitoring, arterial lines of hemodynamically unstable patients, and suctioning and oxygenating. Small groups of three students (100% attendance of class [$n = 49$]) were scheduled outside of class to work in our simulated ICU, partially funded by a Helene Fuld Grant, with the author on a 3:1 student–teacher ratio for practicing with a defibrillator, life pack, simulated monitors, EKG, and pacemaker scenarios in order to get familiar with the equipment on an individualized basis in the beginning of the course.

The Fairfield University School of Nursing's Robin Kanarek Learning Resource Center has several areas for teaching experiential learning. This scenario occurs in the ICU room, which is a simulated one-bed ICU area with cardiac and hemodynamic monitoring, patient chart with medication administration record, ventilator, wall oxygen with hyperventilatory bag, suctioning equipment on a bedside table, and wall suction. There is a high-fidelity HPS in the bed. The director of the Learning Resource Center uses a video recording device to record the scenario so that it can be reused as a debriefing exercise for the larger group of students in the classroom. Using experiential teaching-learning pedagogy to improve student psychomotor abilities as well as communication techniques and critical thinking skills is discussed in this chapter.

C. Course Objectives and Undergraduate Program Terminal Objectives

Course Objectives

Describe the rationale for using basic critical care technology.

Apply therapeutic nursing implications for a variety of case studies of critically ill patients in a holistic manner.

Identify pertinent cues of patients experiencing life-threatening crises who are moving toward a deterioration or recovery of their status.

Describe nursing implications for the classic pharmacologic therapies in caring for critically ill patients.

Discuss ethical, legal, spiritual, and other concerns of patients, families, and caregivers in critical care.

Undergraduate Program Terminal Objectives

Demonstrate effectiveness in planning and providing therapeutic nursing care, managing information, and promoting self-care competence of culturally diverse individuals, families, groups and communities.

Employ a variety of technologies and other therapeutic modalities with sensitivity for the provision of care.

Make sound clinical judgments based on nursing science and related theory using critical thinking and ethical decision making.

Demonstrate collaboration with peers, patient, health care professionals, and others within health care teams in the process of planning, delegating, implementing, and evaluating care.

Communicate with clarity, purpose, and sensitivity using a variety of methods, including technology.

Advocate for patients, consumers, and the nursing profession through involvement in the political process and health/patient care policies and practices.

D. Introduction of Scenario to Include Setting the Scene, Technology Used, Objectives, and Description of Participants

Setting the Scene

Mr. Whisper, an 81-year-old patient, is ventilated and attempting to talk around his endotracheal tube (ET). He is a married, retired judge with a strong Catholic faith. He has three grown children and 12 grandchildren who come to visit regularly. His current diagnosis is chronic obstructive pulmonary disease (COPD) exacerbation (secondary to emphysema) with bilateral lower lobe pneumonia, dyspnea, a long history of atrial fibrillation, coronary artery disease (CAD), hyperlipidemia, and hypertension. He receives lisinopril 10 mg, metoprolol 100 mg, hydroclorothiazide 12.5 mg, a Spiriva inhaler once a day, levofloxacin, warfarin, and fluoxetine. He receives morphine sulfate 2 to 10 mg IV as needed for anxiety. This is his 5th admission to the hospital in 3 months, and his children have brought up the option of "do not resuscitate" (DNR) with him, which he would like, but his wife has been against this option until this admission. He is having multiple high pressure alarm problems due to his emphysema pathology and high amount of mucus plugging from the pneumonia.

When asked a question by the students, he is not strong enough to use a pad but finally is able to maneuver the magic slate with some encouragement. He is oriented to time, place, and situation. He will demonstrate anxiety when he is disconnected from the ventilator for suctioning to remove the mucous plug, and the patient will display isolated unifocal premature ventricular contractions (PVCs). Blood pressure will increase from 128/78 to 170/82 during the suctioning and also when the wife visits. Other relevant data include P: 84, SaO_2, 92%, T: 99.8, RR: 16. He is in atrial fibrillation with an occasional PVC and has a Foley catheter that is draining clear, yellow urine approximately 35 to 40 mL per hour. He has D5 1/2 NS at 75 cc per hour with a left antecubital IV.

Equipment needed includes the following: ventilator, heart monitor, bed, simulated ICU setting, oxygen and suction tubing, suction equipment (both open and closed systems), hyperventilatory bag, oxygen saturation monitor, intravenous supplies (pole, tubing, and bag), Foley catheter in patient, props for wife to wear, intensivist, and nurse giving report.

Technology Used

HPS, cardiac monitor simulator, DVD for use in debriefing, and live real-time video camera recording to a large auditorium for entire class to view.

Objectives

- Communicate with the patient and wife about the patient's condition regarding his palliative care measures.
- Communicate with the nurse giving the previous shift report.
- Demonstrate oral and closed and open ET suctioning and hyperventilation on a ventilated patient.
- Assess breath sounds on a COPD patient with pneumonia.
- Assess PVCs on the patient's cardiac monitor.
- Troubleshoot a ventilated patient with high pressure alarm problems.
- Administer morphine sulfate to an anxious patient according to evidence-based protocols.
- Facilitate the wife's participation with her children and the health care team in a palliative care family meeting, and revise the patient's advanced directives.

National Council Licensure Examination for a Registered Nurse (NCLEX-RN) test plan categories and subcategories (National Council of State Boards of Nursing, 2007) addressed in the simulation are as follows:

Safe and Effective Care Environment
    Management of Care
        Advance Directives
        Collaboration with Interdisciplinary Team
        Delegation
        Establishing Priorities
        Ethical Practice
        Informed Consent
        Legal Rights and Responsibilities
        Resource Management
    Safety and Infection Control
        Medical and Surgical Asepsis
        Standard/Transmission-Based/Other Precautions
        Safe Use of Equipment
Health Promotion and Maintenance
        Aging Process
        Family Systems
        Techniques of Physical Assessment
Psychosocial Integrity
        Coping Mechanisms
        End of Life Care
        Family Dynamics
        Grief and Loss
        Mental Health Concepts
        Religious and Spiritual Influences on Health
        Situational Role Changes
        Support Systems
        Therapeutic Communications
        Unexpected Body Image Changes

Physiological Integrity
> *Basic Care and Comfort*
>> Elimination
>> Nonpharmacological Comfort
>> Palliative/Comfort Care
>> Personal Hygiene
>> Rest and Sleep
>
> *Pharmacological and Parenteral Therapy*
>> Dosage Calculation
>> Expected Effects/Outcomes
>> Medication Administration
>> Parenteral/Intravenous Therapies
>> Pharmacological Agents/Actions
>> Pharmacological Pain Management
>
> *Reduction of Risk Potential*
>> Laboratory Values
>> Potential for Complications of Diagnostic Tests/Treatments/Procedures
>> System Specific Assessments
>> Therapeutic Procedures
>> Vital Signs
>
> *Physiological Adaptation*
>> Hemodynamics
>> Illness Management
>> Medical Emergencies

Description of Participants

Six senior nursing students will work on this scenario and then be peer evaluated. The scenario will be taped, and the real-time enactment will also be shown in the larger classroom. The simulation will be managed by the laboratory director, and there will be one other faculty who will act as the patient's wife, the nurse giving the previous shift report, and the person who will debrief the students.

E. Describe Running of the Scenario

Required Student Assessments and Actions Prior to Running Scenario – Students who have at least two semesters of medical-surgical nursing or are at the end of their second semester should be prepared to successfully manage this scenario. The large course group (e.g., this course has 51 students) will be evaluating their six peers in the auditorium classroom. Students will have been taught the suctioning via ET process (open and closed suction systems), use of ventilator, oral suctioning, hyperventilation, DNR status change policy, and the importance of communication with the patient and family in the lecture part of this course prior to their experience with simulation. Students will be given a copy of the demographics and a detailed report on the patient's behavior the night before. They will be given a report on the patient at the beginning of the scenario. They will have time to ask any questions before the scenario begins and then will discuss their performance and their colleagues' peer evaluation with the faculty and classmates post simulation scenario.

This scenario will take 20 minutes.

F. Presentation of Completed Template

Title: The Older Adult in an ICU with Acute Respiratory Failure

Focus Area:
Nursing 360, Critical Care Nursing, Palliative Care, Medical–Surgical Nursing

Scenario Description:
This chapter focuses on caring for an older adult with COPD who has an exacerbation secondary to pneumonia and who desires full medical treatment, including a ventilator. Simulation practice with students will consist of communication with the patient and his wife regarding palliative versus cure care and skills such as suctioning via an ET with open and closed endotracheal suction systems, oral suction, using a hyperventilation bag and oxygen administration, working with a ventilated patient, and assessment particularly regarding respiratory and cardiac.

Scenario Objectives:
After the completion of this simulated scenario, the students will be able to do the following:

- Communicate with the patient and his wife about the patient's condition regarding his palliative care measures
- Communicate with the nurse giving the previous shift report
- Demonstrate oral and closed and open ET suctioning and hyperventilation on a ventilated patient
- Assess breath sounds on a COPD patient with pneumonia
- Assess PVCs on the patient's cardiac monitor
- Troubleshoot a ventilated patient with high pressure alarm problems
- Administer morphine sulfate to an anxious patient according to evidence-based protocols
- Facilitate the wife's participation with her children and the health care team in a palliative care family meeting and revise the patient's advanced directives

Setting the Scene:

Equipment needed: Ventilator, heart monitor, bed, simulated ICU setting, oxygen and suction tubing, suction equipment (both open and closed systems), hyperventilatory bag, oxygen saturation monitor, intravenous supplies (pole, tubing, and bag), Foley in patient, props for wife to wear, intensivist, and nurse giving report.
Resources needed: Flow sheet, critical care nursing text
Simulator level: Human volunteer(s), HPS

Participants needed: Six students, volunteer to be RN giving report, intensivist, patient's wife (Same person can play all three roles), and person to run HPS and computer

Scenario Implementation:

A simulated ICU cubicle can be created. Student-required actions include taking report, assessing need for medication, Morphine Sulfate, hand washing, patient assessment, administering MS, notifying respiratory therapy and intensivist, creating method of communicating with patient with ET, preoxygenating and hyperventilating patient, suctioning both the ET and orally, assessing patient's EKG monitor, BP, SaO_2, pulse, RR, talking with wife about possible DNR change, assessing patient's needs regarding anxiety and pain/discomfort, and managing an intervention with the intensivist.

Instructor's required interventions include being the RN giving the report, being the intensivist who the student nurses will collaborate with regarding Mr. Whisper's plan, and being Mrs. Whisper. Also, there will be another instructor who runs the HPS and manages the scenario.

Step-By-Step Running of the Scenario:

- Students will be given a report from the "nurse" going off shift. That nurse will say, "I was busier than usual and did not have time to get Mr. Whisper suctioned in the last 3 hours. He needs some help now that he is agitated with the ET and the high pressure ventilator alarm has been triggered. I am not having success communicating with him, and his wife is not satisfied with his care. She was in last evening and was complaining to the second-shift nurse, who told me that the wife and children are going to have a family meeting regarding possibly changing Mr. Whisper's DNR status. He has not had MS for more than 6 hours."
- After the report, the students will check the medication documentation and prepare the MS for administration.
- Students will make an introduction to the patient, who is trying to talk. Students will give him a pad, and some effective communication will transpire.
- Students will assess Mr. Whisper and determine how much MS he should receive and give it. He should receive 8 mg IV push.
- Students will see that he needs immediate suctioning, since the high pressure alarm is triggering every 2 to 3 minutes and the airway pressure is >40 cm H_2O.
- Students will preoxygenate him via the ventilator with 100% O_2 and begin closed suctioning but will be unsuccessful in suctioning enough of the mucus to shut off the alarm. Students will stop and decrease the FiO_2 back to 40%, as it was previously set at the 100% setting.
- Students will auscultate Mr. Whisper's lungs and determine decreased breath sounds in the LLL and rhonchi. (This is a deterioration, as previously he was clearing in both left and right lung fields.) Students will notice PVCs on the monitor, and the SaO_2 will decrease to low 80s from 91.
- At this time, students will determine that Mr. Whisper is agitated and is trying to talk around his ET, his respiratory rate is 36 breaths per minute,

he is fighting the ventilator, and the high pressure alarm is almost constantly alarming since the airway pressure is around 50 cm H_2O.

■ The wife will arrive and become hysterical about her husband's inability to catch his breath and the alarming ventilator. She will say, "My husband is a judge, and he needs to be treated with utmost dignity. He cannot be allowed to feel that he cannot catch his breath. What are you doing? You look so unprepared. I am going to get a nurse who knows how to care for him. You are just unfit, and why are so many of you in here bothering him?"

■ One student will take the wife away from the patient and discuss the situation with her as well as their plan to remove the plug so that he will stop alarming the high pressure alarm. Students will have a discussion about the upcoming family conference about changing to DNR status.

■ Students will explain to the patient their plan of removing him from the ventilator to suction him. Students will take the patient off the ventilator and use the hyperventilatory bag to administer 100% O_2 and three large, deep breaths. Students will suction his ET three times and procure the mucous plug along with large amounts of mucus. Students note that there are approximately 4 PVCs per minute, and this is increasing. Students will orally suction him and simultaneously bag the patient with oxygenated breaths. Students will reattach to the ventilator. Students will note that the PVCs have decreased to one PVC every 4 or 5 minutes since oxygenating him so patient does not need any antiarrhythmic drugs.

■ Students will collaborate with the ICU intensivist, who is rounding at this time regarding the need for increased suctioning, more mucolytics, and more scheduled MS administration. Students will record they gave the MS 8 mg. (Asking the students what areas—suctioning, oxygenating, using ventilator, medicating, respiratory assessment, communicating with the family, assessing EKG, and monitoring vital signs.)

This process is written using evidence-based data from a meta-analysis of open and closed endotracheal suction study (Jongerden, Rovers, & Grypdonck, & Bonten, 2007).

Evaluative Criteria:
The following are required student assessment and performance actions:

_____ Receive report from the previous shift nurse—ask if last suctioning 3 hours ago was productive.

_____ Assess documentation in Medication Administration Record regarding MS administration.

_____ Wash hands.

_____ Prepare MS 10 mg cartridge to administer to Mr. Whisper (order says that 2 to 10 mg IV push prn may be given).

_____ Wash hands.

_____ Introduce self to patient—establish communication method with Mr. Whisper.

_____ Assess patient vital signs, respiratory exam, rhythm strip, and ventilator airway pressure.

_____ Give 8 mg of MS IV and flush line with saline.

_____ Talking with Mr. Whisper while preparing the suction equipment and explaining to him what is going to be done to stop the high pressure alarm and make him feel better.

_____ Preoxygenate with 100% O_2 by pushing this setting on the ventilator and then closed suctioning will occur.

_____ Assessment of the airway pressure gauge shows a decrease, but not low enough, and the alarm is still alarming. The SaO_2 is decreasing to low 80s, and respiratory assessment indicates rhonchi and LLL decreased breath sounds.

_____ Continue closed suctioning with the patient's head and trunk turned toward the right side to improve the possibility of getting down the left bronchi. There is some improvement, but there still is a need for a more aggressive technique.

_____ Prepare the open suctioning equipment and hyperventilatory bag and connect to 100% O_2.

_____ Reset the O_2 setting to 40% on the ventilator.

_____ Detach the ET from the ventilator.

_____ Attach the hyperventilatory bag, and deliver three hyperinflation breaths.

_____ Suction via the ET and returns will indicate thicker mucus being removed than with the closed suctioning. Note the PVCs, and note that they stop when O_2 reapplied in between suctioning passes.

_____ Suction orally.

_____ Reattach the ET to the ventilator.

_____ Respiratory assessment indicates clear breath sounds on the left and right side.

_____ Talk with Mr. Whisper who is using his slate and is quite comfortable now with SaO_2 at 91, RR at 16, and airway pressure at 22 cm H_2O.

_____ Mrs. Whisper has completed her discussion with the other nurse and wants reinforcement that she is doing the "right" thing by choosing a DNR status for her husband.

_____ Mr. Whisper thanks the nurse and says, "I have not felt this good about my breathing since midnight."

_____ Reassure the patient that he will continue to have heavy secretions and that they will be suctioned out frequently.

_____ Answer any questions from Mr. or Mrs. Whisper.

_____ Chart administration of MS.

_____ Set up a discussion with the intensivist regarding the necessity of hourly suctioning, increased frequency of MS administration, and the need to encourage Mrs. Whisper and family to honor Mr. Whisper's wishes of setting up a DNR order.

G. Debriefing Guidelines

The instructor reviews the evaluative criteria with rationales with the six students and entire group (Augustyn, 2007; Neil-Weise, Snoeren, & van den Broek, 2007; Ruffell & Adamcova, 2008; Jongerden et al., 2007). The following questions should be covered:

1. How did you prepare for your participation in this scenario?
2. What references did you use?
3. If you could go back in time, what would you have said to the nurse reporting off to you about how she did not suction Mr. Whisper since her workload was so high and she was so focused on the bowel movement?
4. Did you feel prepared to manage the mucous plug with Mr. Whisper?
5. How did you think you demonstrated your suctioning skills with the ET? Orally?
6. How did you feel you communicated with Mr. Whisper, who cannot talk with his ET?
7. Did you feel comfortable giving the additional MS?
8. Did you feel comfortable assessing the airway pressure and using the ventilator to preoxygenate and hyperventilate with the hyperventilatory bag?
9. How do you perceive you succeeded with your talk with Mrs. Whisper about possibly making her husband a DNR?
10. Did you and the other students collaborate well with the intensivist?

Also, the students who did not participate are asked to assess their peers' performance.

H. Suggestions/Key Features to Replicate or Improve

Being able to actually practice with instructor feedback in a college laboratory prior to integrating the whole scenario with the HPS has improved skills greatly in the scenario. It is suggested that lecture with demonstration be first given to the students regarding the skills associated with this scenario. Without giving the students all the hints regarding caring for this type of patient in the class, teach them about the skills and how they relate to the patient's condition. Next, offer a college laboratory practice session where each student gets to demonstrate his or her skill with closed and open suctioning. As well, if the students have not had advanced directive content, this also needs to be discussed. By allowing each student an opportunity to practice the skill individually and then integrating the skills into a scenario such as that with Mr. Whisper, the students have more confidence in their ability to manage a patient desaturation with mucous plug situation in combination with the communication with the wife.

I. Recommendations for Further Use

This simulation is applicable for use in practicing and evaluating communication skills regarding the anxious wife who is trying to decide about her husband's DNR status, communicating with a ventilated patient, and collaborating with the intensivist and other members of the health care team regarding family decision making about advanced directives. This example could be focused on communication, and the suctioning and high pressure alarm situation could be completely deleted. The HPS, Mr. Whisper, could just be quiet and not be experiencing any desaturation.

Also, this simulated scenario could be broken into parts where the educator can teach just the ventilator and alarms with a high focus on pressure alarms and the main settings of FiO_2, mode, PEEP, frequency, tidal volume, and airway pressure. Or, the educator could just focus on the suctioning since there are three separate types of suctioning in this scenario: (1) oral suctioning, (2) closed suctioning of ET, and (3) open suctioning of ET. Additionally, this scenario offers the use of a hyperventilatory bag and oxygenation of a ventilated patient.

As presented, this scenario is in a capstone course focusing on critically ill patients, so it offers multiple challenging learning experiences to senior students.

J. Discussion of Simulation-Based Pedagogy and How This New Technology Has Contributed to Improved Student Outcomes

Student satisfaction with their learning increases if they are able to carry out the skills involved in a safe, simulated setting prior to performing these same skills on real patients. Rather than expecting competent performance from students without prior practice, more successful outcomes are expected when the students have had time to practice skills at their own pace and with guidance. Complicated patient situations that require excellent communication skills and savvy in administering high technologic skills in a life-threatening situation are challenging to experienced RNs. So, it is only reasonable to assume that students should have opportunities to practice in a simulated environment prior to having to perform with real patients. Students have evaluated this type of teaching as paramount to increasing the effectiveness of their learning (Waldner & Olson, 2007).

References

Augustyn, B. (2007). Ventilator-associated pneumonia: Risk factors and management. *Critical Care Nurse, 27*(4), 32–39.

Jongerden, I., Rovers, M., Grypdonck, M., & Bonten, M. (2007). Open and closed endotracheal suction systems in mechanically ventilated intensive care patients: A meta-analysis. *Critical Care Medicine, 35*(1), 260–270.

National Council of State Boards of Nursing. (2007). *NCLEX-RN examination: Test plan for the National Council Licensure Examination for Registered Nurses.* Retrieved December 3, 2007, from https://www.ncsbn.org/RN_Test_Plan_2007_Web.pdf

Neil-Weise, B. S., Snoeren, R. L. M., & van den Broek, P. J. (2007). Policies for endotracheal suctioning of patients receiving mechanical ventilation: A systematic review of randomized controlled trials. *Infection Control and Hospital Epidemiology, 28*(5), 531–536.

Ruffell, A., & Adamcova, L. (2008). Ventilator-associated pneumonia: Prevention is better than cure. *Nursing in Critical Care, 13*(1), 44–53.

Waldner, M. H., & Olson, J. K. (2007). Taking the patient to the classroom: Applying theoretical frameworks to simulation in nursing education. *International Journal of Nursing Education Scholarship, 4*(1), Article 18.

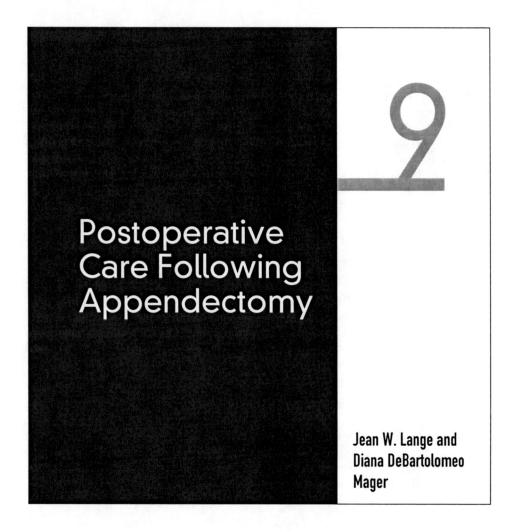

Postoperative Care Following Appendectomy

Jean W. Lange and
Diana DeBartolomeo
Mager

A. Discussion of Implementation of Simulation-Based Pedagogy in Each Contributor's Individualized Teaching

This chapter will incorporate student knowledge of postsurgical patients, with an emphasis on postoperative assessment, problem recognition, interdisciplinary collaboration, and patient teaching for prevention of postoperative complications.

Although I (Dr. Lange) had attended several workshops and demonstrations about how to conduct a simulated scenario, this scenario was my first. Few if any of our faculty had used a scenario in front of students at this point, and we all felt a bit intimidated. Students conveyed to faculty that they were anxious to experience simulations now that we had our first human patient simulator (HPS) on the premises. This feedback gave us the impetus that faculty needed to forge ahead. Our lab director, Diana D. Mager, initiated the process by sending an e-mail to several faculty members suggesting that we collectively create a simple scenario. She suggested that we begin with a postoperative patient in pain. As the medical-surgical faculty, I quickly saw the possible fit with my junior medical-surgical course, where postoperative care is taught. Through several back-and-forth e-mails, we began to fill in more details for the scenario. Objectives and a checklist of desired student activities quickly followed. The scenario was scheduled during class, with three faculty in attendance: our lab director, the course faculty, and our faculty champion of simulation integration. Working together decreased our anxiety about "going alone" and freed the course faculty to facilitate the scenario while others served as the "handler" or as the patient's "on-call" health care provider.

B. Description of Educational Materials Available in Your Teaching Area and Relative to Your Specialty

At Fairfield University, the School of Nursing's Robin Kanarek Learning Resource Center was developed in 2006 to include an area designated for acute-care simulations. One room is designed to simulate either an intensive care area or a private room on a medical-surgical unit. Items mounted on the walls include the following:

- Working oxygen/suction headwall unit
- X-ray screen
- Hand sanitizer
- Sharps container with glove dispenser
- Large flat-screen monitor that can project images or lab values sent in from the adjacent control room

Portable equipment housed in the room includes the following:

- High-fidelity human patient simulator (HPS) in a hospital bed
- Intravenous pumps on poles
- Stryker stretcher
- Ventilator
- ECG machine
- Rolling vital signs station
- Wheelchair
- Linen cart
- Overbed table

In addition, cabinets house various props, supplies, and equipment that may be used for any patient care needed during a simulation.

One wall of the ICU simulation area abuts a control room, where a handler can control the high-fidelity HPS without students in the ICU seeing him or her. A double-sided mirror is used so that the instructor can see all that is going on in the simulation, yet students are not distracted by seeing the instructor. While in the control room, the handler can communicate via microphone to students in the simulation area. In addition, while a simulation is occurring, the whole episode can be projected into nearby larger classrooms for viewing in real time. The simulation can also be recorded from the control room for future use.

C. Specific Objective for Simulation Utilization Within a Specific Course and the Overall Program

The primary objective of this scenario is to assess the student's ability to conduct a thorough postoperative assessment, recognize abnormal findings, and cluster cues to diagnose actual and potential problems. Elements of interdisciplinary collaboration, infection control, communication skills, and judgment in medication administration are incorporated. This scenario was designed as an in-class introductory simulation for junior nursing students taking their first medical-surgical nursing course. Students have previously completed coursework in pathophysiology, pharmacology, technical skills, and physical assessment. Although students have had clinical experiences in long-term care and in the community, they have had minimal exposure to acute-care settings. This simulation early in the course follows content on postoperative care and provides an opportunity to practice a head-to-toe assessment before entering the hospital.

D. Introduction of Scenario to Include Setting the Scene, Technology Used, Objectives, and Description of Participants

The patient is a 54-year-old man who presented to the emergency room with a diagnosis of appendicitis. The students arrive at the surgical unit of the hospital for clinical the next morning. The students learn from the night nurse's report that the patient had an appendectomy the previous evening.

E. Describe Running of the Scenario

Prior to the scenario, a HPS was prepared by setting the various findings that would be pertinent for students to assess for a postoperative patient. Initial vital signs (BP: 144/94, P: 98, RR: 20, T: 98.9), lung sounds (slightly diminished bilaterally), and bowel sounds (hypoactive) were determined and preset. A wound with a Penrose drain was placed on the right lower quadrant with a dressing in place that contained a small amount of red drainage simulated by food coloring. A wristband with the patient name and an allergy alert to morphine was placed on the wrist. An IV bag of D5NS was set up and attached to the arm. Stethoscopes, gloves, and a pulse oximeter were placed nearby for student use. As the students approached the patient, he was groaning and grimacing. As students asked the patient questions, answers were given via preset verbal options. When students asked for further information about the patient, one of the faculty members would answer their requests as though they were medical personnel on the unit. The scenario lasted approximately 10 minutes, not including the period of debriefing.

F. Presentation of Completed Template

Title: Postoperative Care Following Appendectomy

Focus Area:
NS 312: Patterns of Illness I: First Medical-surgical nursing course, junior year

Scenario Description:
The students are arriving at 7 a.m. for clinical at an acute-care surgical unit. The students are assigned to care for Joshua Rivera. The night nurse gives the following report:

> *Patient:* Mr. Joshua Rivera
> *Age:* 53 years
> *Allergies:* Morphine
> *History:* Hypertension; 12 hours post appendectomy

Joshua Rivera is a 54-year-old patient of Dr. Lange's with a history of hypertension. He came into the emergency room yesterday morning complaining of severe abdominal pain and a high fever. He was diagnosed with appendicitis and had an appendectomy late yesterday morning. Mr. Rivera slept through the night, and his vital signs have been stable. His dressing is dry and intact. He has an IV of D5NS running at 75 mL per hour and is on a clear liquid diet. He has tolerated a glass of water and some apple juice so far. His only medication is a blood pressure pill, but he can have morphine for pain if needed. He has not requested any pain medication.

Scenario Objectives:

1. Introduce self and role in the patient's care.
2. Complete a thorough postoperative assessment.
3. Observe universal precautions.
4. Cluster cues to diagnose actual and potential patient problems (e.g., relate increased BP and HR to pain; recognize pain as a deterrent to cough, deep breathing, and mobility).
5. Access interdisciplinary team resources when needed (e.g., calls health care provider regarding morphine allergy).
6. Conduct teaching to prevent postoperative complications following abdominal surgery.

For this scenario, the National Council of State Boards of Nursing's (2007) RN test plan categories addressed are as follows:

Safe and Effective Care Environment
    Management of Care
        Advocacy
        Collaboration With Interdisciplinary Team
        Establishing Priorities
    Safety and Infection Control
        Error Prevention
Health Promotion and Maintenance
        Principles of Teaching/Learning
        Techniques of Physical Assessment
Psychosocial Integrity
        Cultural Diversity
Physiological Integrity
    Basic Care and Comfort
        Elimination
        Mobility/Immobility
        Non-pharmacological Comfort Interventions
        Nutrition and Oral Hydration
    Pharmacological and Parenteral Therapies
        Adverse Effects/Contraindications
        Parenteral/Intravenous Therapies
        Pharmacological Agents/Actions
        Pharmacological Pain Management
    Reduction of Risk Potential
        Laboratory Values
        Potential for Alterations in Body Systems
        Potential for Complications from Surgical Procedures and Health
          Alterations
        System Specific Assessments
        Vital Signs
    Physiological Adaptation
        Pathophysiology

Setting the Scene:

Equipment needed:

- High-fidelity HPS on gurney or bed
- Video recording device (optional)
- Projection screen (optional)
- Pulse oximeter
- Allergy bracelet with morphine listed
- Penrose drain with dressing
- Incentive spirometer
- Gloves
- D5NS intravenous setup
- BP cuff and stethoscopes
- I & O record

Resources needed:

- Student activity checklist
- Medication record (copy the following medication card for students to use during the scenario)

Patient: Mr. Joshua Rivera	**Allergy:** Morphine
DOB: 2/21/53	**Medical Provider:** J. Lange, M.D.

Medication List:	**Time Due:**
Metoprolol (Lopressor) 100 mg po daily	09:00
Multivitamin 1 tab po q am	09:00
Docusate sodium (Colace) 100 mg po q am	09:00

PRN List:	**Time Given:**
Morphine sulfate IV 6–10 mg every 4 hours prn for severe pain	
Hydrocodone–acetaminophen (Percocet) 1–2 tabs po every 4 hours prn pain	
Acetaminophen (Tylenol) 2 tabs po prn Temp >101°F	
Promethazine (Phenergan) 10–25 mg im every 4 hours prn nausea	

Participant roles:

- Handler will change settings in response to student actions and speak for the patient in response to student questions.
- Student will role-play the night nurse delivering report.
- Faculty can serve as the health care provider on call or the nurse caring for the patient on the unit during the day shift and also record student actions on the checklist.
- Up to four students may share the care of Mr. Rivera.

Scenario Implementation

Initial Settings

- Apply wrist band with allergy alert to morphine sulfate.
- Make a print out of medications available to students on request.
- Simulate facial grimacing on the manikin.
- Project monitor readings onto a large screen (optional).
- Set for hypoactive bowel sounds and slightly decreased breath sounds.
- Apply Penrose drain covered with a dressing showing sanguinous drainage to right lower quadrant.

Required Student Assessments and Actions

- Wash hands.
- Introduce self.
- Check name band.
- Note allergy to morphine.
- Assess general condition.
- Check IV site, solution, and rate.
- Assess vital signs and pulse oximetry.
- Note abnormal BP and rechecks BP.
- Auscultate lungs and notes diminished breath sounds.
- Palpate pulses/checks capillary refill.
- Don gloves to observe dressing/wound.
- Auscultate bowel sounds.
- Note decreased bowel sounds.
- Ask patient if experiencing nausea/vomiting, moved bowels, or passed flatus postoperatively.
- Ask if urinating.
- Check I & O sheet.
- Assess ambulation status (has patient been out of bed?).
- Determine need for a.m. medication (BP medication)
- Determine need for pain medication.
- Notice allergy to the medication ordered.
- Call health care provider about morphine allergy.
- Give Percocet.
- Recheck BP after medications are administered.
- Evaluate response to pain medication (scale of 1-10).
- Complete teaching regarding preventing postoperative complications.

Instructor Interventions

- Debriefing

Evaluation Criteria:

Checklist of Interventions and Assessments

- _____ Wash hands.
- _____ Introduce self.
- _____ Check name band
- _____ Note allergy to morphine.
- _____ Ask how patient is doing.
- _____ Ask about pain level on 1 to 10 scale.
- _____ Check IV for proper fluid and rate.
- _____ Check IV site.
- _____ Assess vital signs.
  - _____ BP
  - _____ P
  - _____ RR
  - _____ Temp
  - _____ Pulse oximetry

_____ Find abnormal BP.
_____ Recheck BP if found abnormal.
_____ Auscultate lungs.
_____ Find decreased breath sounds.
_____ Palpate pulses/checks capillary refill.
_____ Don gloves.
_____ Observe dressing/wound.
_____ Auscultate bowel sounds.
_____ Note decreased bowel sounds.
_____ Ask patient if experiencing any nausea/vomiting.
_____ Ask patient if moved bowels or passed flatus postoperatively.
_____ Ask if urinating.
_____ Check I & O sheet.
_____ Assess ambulation status (has patient been out of bed?).
_____ Determine need for a.m. medication (BP medication).
_____ Determine need for pain medication.
_____ Notice allergy to medication.
_____ Call Dr. Lange about morphine allergy.
_____ Give Percocet.
_____ Recheck BP after medications are administered.
_____ Evaluate response to pain medication (scale of 1–10).
_____ Complete teaching regarding preventing postoperative complications:
        _____ Cough, turn, deep breath
        _____ Use of incentive spirometry
        _____ Splinting
        _____ Importance of early ambulation
        _____ Importance of pain management

G. Debriefing Guidelines

1. What challenges did you face?
2. Would you do anything differently next time?
3. What problems/nursing diagnoses did you identify for this patient (e.g., pain, risk for ineffective breathing pattern/infection, potential for altered elimination [GI], allergy)?
4. What nursing interventions would be appropriate?
5. What additional information would you have liked to have in the report?
6. Are there any lab results you would like to see?

H. Suggestions/Key Features to Replicate or Improve

■ This was students' first exposure to a simulation experience; therefore, they were unfamiliar with its idiosyncrasies (e.g., where to listen to lung sounds, where to place the stethoscope to auscultate a blood pressure, where pulses can be felt).

- Faculty learned a few "tricks" that have aided students' ability to recognize planned abnormalities (e.g., turning the breath sounds and pulse volumes up high to facilitate hearing crackles and Korotkoff sounds).
- Students ideally should have an orientation to simulation before using it in a live scenario. We now do this in health assessment.
- We did not make copies of the scenario (report, patient information, medication list) for the class ahead of time. In retrospect, this would have been helpful.
- Use of preset verbal options to answer student questions was of limited benefit. It took too long to find appropriate answers, and answers to specific questions were not always available. The scenario would have been more realistic with use of a microphone to enable the person running the scenario to actually speak for the simulator.

I. Recommendations for Further Use

More complexity can be added as students become more familiar with the medical surgical content related to postoperative patients, and as faculty who run the scenarios become more familiar with the simulators. In this scenario, the patient was allergic to the pain medication ordered. One strategy to incorporate interdisciplinary collaboration could be expecting the student to contact the physician or other provider to change the medication order. Postoperative complications could also be added to the scenario (e.g., urinary retention, constipation, infection, ileus, etc.).

J. Discussion of Simulation-Based Pedagogy and How This New Technology Has Contributed to Improved Student Outcomes

- Start with a simple scenario having only one or two objectives.
- Work in teams to develop and conduct scenarios.
- Practice the scenario on colleagues before using it with students.
- Checklists of desired student activities can be a useful alternative if you have not yet mastered scenario programming or want to use simulation on short notice. They are easy for faculty to track key behaviors that students do or forget to do during the scenario and are a useful resource during debriefing.
- To keep students engaged that are not participating in the scenario, ask them to write questions or suggestions as they watch the scenario unfold.
- When debriefing in front of a class, allow the students who participated in the scenario to critique themselves first. This decreases feelings of being judged by their peers. Other students can then share their questions and suggestions with the class.

Reference

National Council of State Boards of Nursing. (2007). *NCLEX-RN examination: Test plan for the National Council Licensure Examination for Registered Nurses.* Retrieved June 18, 2008, from https://www.ncsbn.org/RN_Test_Plan_2007_Web.pdf

Recommended Text

Lewis, S. M., Heitkemper, M. M., Dirksen, S. R., O'Brien, P. G., & Bucher, L. (2007). *Medical-surgical nursing: Assessment and management of clinical problems* (7th ed.). St Louis: Mosby.

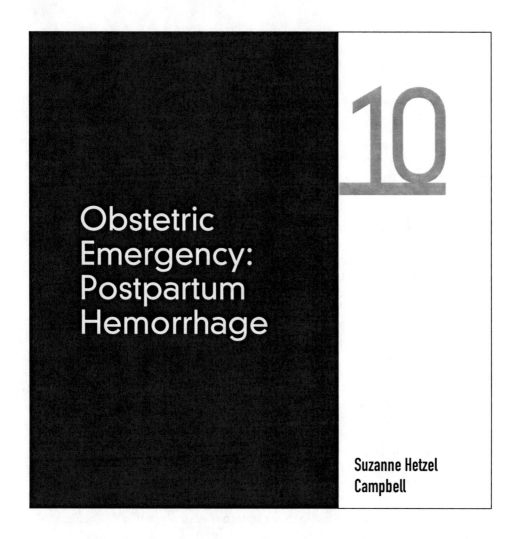

10

Obstetric Emergency: Postpartum Hemorrhage

Suzanne Hetzel Campbell

A. Discussion of Implementation of Simulation-Based Pedagogy in Each Contributor's Individualized Teaching

Experiences for the obstetric and pediatric clinical areas are becoming difficult to acquire for students, as increasing numbers of students compete for a small number of slots and constraints on numbers of students allowed into the areas continues to rise. For example, 8 to 10 students may be placed on a large medical floor with one instructor. In contrast, most of the family birthing units limit the number of students allowed to six, perhaps a maximum of eight. Add to this that students need to rotate through at least three different areas—postpartum, intrapartum (labor and delivery), and newborn nursery (or neonatal ICU)—and this adds to the complexity of scheduling and student education. Students must be prepared early on for the varied assessments and unique skills required for all the areas.

Presently, simulation-based pedagogy has been implemented in this area with the use of an intermediate-fidelity pregnant human patient simulator (HPS) to demonstrate Leopold maneuvers, fundal height measurement, infant positioning in utero (e.g., for placement of external fetal monitors and to monitor the birth process), and in some cases the birth process. Other potentialities for the use of this model include the demonstration and practice of obstetric emergencies such as shoulder dystocia, prolapsed umbilical cord, placenta previa, and abruptio placenta.

Basic skills for clinical orientation to this rotation are set up as a clinical orientation day. The stations for student education and practice include several models.

Newborn infant static HPS allows:
- Newborn assessment
- Newborn bath, cord care, vitamin K and hepatitis B injections
- Newborn blood draw for indications of genetic disorders such as PKU, maple syrup urine disease, and so forth (newborn foot, alcohol wipe, lancet, etc.)
- Formula preparation and provision
- Breast-feeding positioning and practice (breast-feeding doll with breast, such as Lactessa)

Intermediate-fidelity pregnant HPS allows:
- Leopold maneuvers, assessment of infant positioning, FHR monitoring, comfort techniques and positioning for labor

Medium-fidelity HPS allows:
- Postpartum assessment (vaginal and abdominal delivery [cesarean section], fundal check with option for boggy or firm fundus and ability to displace location)
- Postpartum care (perineal care, breast care)

The clinical orientation using these stations is usually run in a 3-hour period with one faculty in charge of one general area and five to seven students per group. Each area lasts about one-half hour and is set up with materials the day before. In addition, a newborn physical exam and gestational age exam video are shown (about 25 minutes each). The clinical packet with written materials for the course is shared and reviewed with the students at this time. After the 3-hour clinical orientation, students meet their clinical faculty for a hospital orientation, including getting identification badges, learning the computer systems, hospital safety, confidentiality, and infant abduction policies at their respective institutions. All the paperwork is completed at this time, and this is the students' full "clinical day." From that point on, they are taking assignments and working with patients while under faculty and staff guidance for six more weeks. This orientation focuses on normal patients, thus scenarios for this area tend to focus on at-risk situations.

B. Description of Educational Materials Available in Your Teaching Area and Relative to Your Specialty

The Fairfield University School of Nursing's Robin Kanarek Learning Resource Center, developed in 2006, has two designated "acute-care settings." With funding from the Connecticut Health and Education Facilities Authority (2007) grant for a "Women's Health Expansion Project," a new area specific to the needs of this clinical specialty will be in place within the year (see chapters 3 and 25). At present, the postpartum hemorrhage scenario takes place in the acute-care area using a high-fidelity HPS. A control room is adjacent with a view into the simulation room through mirrored glass, and the scenario can be projected live via a 360-degree camera into one of two larger classrooms (seating 35 and 90+ students, respectively). Faculty can communicate with students in the simulation room in one of three ways: (1) via a microphone into the room, (2) via a microphone from the high-fidelity HPS, and (3) via phone (e.g., as a doctor or call to unit desk, etc.). Shortly, an electronic medical system will be added and accessible by a computer on wheels (see chapter 25). Finally, the scenario can be DVD recorded from the control room for debriefing and student evaluation/assessment.

C. Specific Objective for Simulation Utilization Within a Specific Course and the Overall Program

The primary objective of this scenario is to assess the students' ability to conduct a thorough postpartum assessment, recognize abnormal findings, and act to determine a plan of action to enhance patient safety and emotional stability. This scenario was designed as an in-class, advanced-level simulation for third-year baccalaureate or first-year associate degree nursing students in their second semester. Students will be taking a medical-surgical course concurrently and have completed pathophysiology, pharmacology, technical skills, and physical assessment courses. This scenario would take place midway through the semester, when the students have had some exposure to this specialty clinical area. Most will have had at least one experience in labor and delivery and/or postpartum and will have completed a postpartum assessment.

Student Learning Activities

- Review and practice normal postpartum assessment.
- Review risk factors for postpartum complications.
- Review medications: pain, oxytocics, postpartum.

D. Introduction of Scenario to Include Setting the Scene, Technology Used, Objectives, and Description of Participants

Setting the Scene

The setting is a hospital room on a postpartum unit of a tertiary-level institution. The students receive report from the night nurse, a certified nurse-midwife is available on call, and the infant is in the neonatal ICU being observed for hypoglycemia.

Technology Used

The medium-fidelity HPS is a female (red wig—increased risk of hemorrhage in redheads and genitalia in place), running manually, with initially normal vital signs (BP: 90/60, P: 100, RR: 16, T: 98.5), but these do not show on the monitor, and the pulse oximeter is not in place. The patient has a saline lock on from IV antibiotics in labor for group B streptococcus–positive status. She is wearing a pad with gauze panties that is soaked through with two plum-sized clots (paste and food coloring). A boggy uterus displaced to the right will be present in the medium-fidelity HPS using a fundal model. A wristband identifies the patient as "Mrs. Althea Jones." Stethoscopes, gloves, and a pulse oximeter are placed nearby for student use, as well as: IV fluids (choices of 1,000 mL D5NS, Ringer, or normal saline), tubing, and blood products. Clean perineal pads, gauze panties, and a pericare bottle are nearby. Routine and as-needed (prn) medications are available (Davidson, London, & Ladewig, 2008, p. 1160):

- Oxytocin (Pitocin, Syntocinon) 10–20 U im. The patient has a saline lock, so oxytocin may be given IV. You would have a main IV, and the oxytocin would be put into the lowest port on the main IV tubing
- Methylergonovine maleate (Methergine) 0.2 mg im q 2–4 hours (contraindicated labile BP or hypertension or cardiac disease, five doses max)
- Ergonovine maleate (Ergotrate Maleate) 0.2 mg im every 2–4 hours (contraindicated labile BP or hypertension, five dose max)
- Analgesics for uterine cramping discomfort (Percocet 1–2 tabs every 3–4 hours; ibuprofen 600 mg every 6 hours)

Objectives

1. Describe the assessment of the woman who is at risk for postpartum complications.
2. Incorporate preventive measures in the care of the postpartal woman specifically at risk for postpartum hemorrhage.
3. Obtain a history to determine if there is a predisposition to hemorrhage.
4. Examine labor and delivery history to identify risk for hemorrhage.
5. Perform an accurate postpartum assessment.
6. Educate patient regarding her status and on normal findings.
7. Determine religious preference to establish if blood transfusions will be permitted.

Description of Participants

Mrs. Althea Jones: 35-year-old white woman. Obstetric history includes gravida 4, term 3, preterm 1, abortions 1, living 3. Came in for augmentation of labor with pitocin Saturday morning. Had a vacuum-assisted delivery of 9 lb 8 oz male on Sunday at 3:07 a.m.; long labor—difficult delivery, pushed for longer than 1 hour. Notice that membranes ruptured Friday evening. Certified Nurse-Midwife (CNM) Robinson is on call for care of Mrs. Jones, who is a clinic patient.

E. Describe Running of the Scenario

Students come into the simulation room and are given the above history. They are told it is Monday morning, and they are finding Mrs. Jones diaphoretic, feverish, and with tachycardia and a falling blood pressure. The goal is for the students to pick up on the risk factors from the patient history. Based on the vital signs, they should quickly perform a postpartum check and find the boggy and displaced fundus as well as lochia soaking the pad with large-size clots. Priority care will involve calling for help, running IV fluids with oxytocin, and performing fundal massage. They should recognize the potential for blood transfusions and surgery dependent on the cause for bleeding.

F. Presentation of Completed Template

Title: Obstetric Emergency: Postpartum Hemorrhage

Focus Area:
Nursing 314: Nursing Care of Women and the Childbearing Family, specialty clinical course in obstetrics for second-semester third-year baccalaureate or first-year associate degree nursing students.

Scenario Description:
The students arrive at 7 a.m. for clinical at a tertiary-level institution on the family birthing unit floor in postpartum. They are assigned to care for Mrs. Althea Jones, a clinic patient being overseen by Ms. Robinson, CNM. The infant is under the care of Mr. Philips, a pediatric nurse practitioner (PNP), and presently is in the neonatal ICU. The night nurse gives the following report:

Patient: Mrs. Althea Jones (A.J.)
Age: 35 years
DOB: 01/20/1973
Allergies: NKDA
History: Gravida 4, term 3, preterm 1, abortions 1, living 3 and now new 9 lb 8 oz male on Sunday at 3:07 a.m. Breast-feeding, infant latched after delivery but was being observed for hypoglycemia and has not been in since midnight. Children at home are 6, 4, and 2 years old, two girls and a boy, respectively. Husband was present for birth but headed home to care for other children.
Delivery history: Augmentation of labor with pitocin early Saturday morning; vacuum-assisted delivery; long labor—difficult delivery, pushed >1 hour. Membranes ruptured Friday evening. At midnight, vital signs (BP: 90/60, P: 100, RR: 16, T: 98.5); HgB 12.0, Hct 35% at admission. The patient has a saline lock from IV antibiotics in labor for group B strep–positive status (received amoxicillin 1 amp X3), 18-gauge needle is in place. Her fundus has been firm, midline, one fingerbreadth above umbilicus, lochia rubra, moderate amount, report was that episiotomy with 4th-degree laceration was fine when transferred to floor.

When students enter room, this is what they find:

- Monday morning VS: BP: 65/45, P: 120, RR: 16 to 20, T: 101.
- Fundus: Boggy and displaced to right of umbilicus.
- Lochia: Bright red, pad soaked with two plum-size clots; question slight odor.
- Episiotomy with 4th-degree laceration: R-2, E-2, E-3, D-3, A-1 = 11; no signs of cervical lacerations, hematoma, or other problems.
- A.J. complains of dizziness, color is pale, slight diaphoresis noticed on forehead. She also is very tender to palpation of uterus and complains of a slight backache.
- A.J. is not hungry and is very teary. Lab values: Group B strep +; VDRL neg; HIV neg; WBC 80,000, HgB 9.7; Hct 30% (10% change from admission), blood type O+ (two units cross matched and on hold).

Medication Record

Patient: Mrs. Althea Jones   **Allergy:** NKDA

DOB: 01/20/1973   **Medical Provider:** Ms. Robinson, CNM

Notes: Nothing per rectum

Medication List:	Time Given:
Docusate sodium (Colace) 100 mg po bid	08:00/20:00
Multivitamin 1 tab po q am	08:00

PRN List: **Time Given:**

Oxytocin (Pitocin, Syntocinon) 10–20 U im; 1 dose prn heavy bleeding

Methylergonovine maleate (Methergine) 0.2 mg im every 2–4 hours prn heavy bleeding (hold with BP >140/90 or cardiac disease, 5 doses max)

Ergonovine maleate (Ergotrate Maleate) 0.2 mg im every 2–4 hours prn heavy bleeding (hold with BP >140/90, 5 dose max);

Hydrocodone-Acetaminophen (Percocet) 1 to 2 tabs po every 3–4 hours prn pain

Ibuprofen (Motrin) 600 mg po every 6 hours prn pain

Scenario Objectives:

1. Students introduce themselves to the patient, check name band, get information about present status, and explain exam to be performed.
2. Obtain a history to determine if there is a predisposition to hemorrhage. Risk factors include but are not limited to maternal history of preeclampsia/eclampsia, previous hemorrhage; uterine overdistention (multiple gestation, polyhydramnios, or large infant—macrosomia); grandmultiparity. (*Debriefing:* This patient is a grandmultip, 4th pregnancy, large infant, long labor, difficult delivery.)

3. Examine labor and delivery history to identify risk for hemorrhage, including augmentation or induction of labor (oxytocin use); dysfunctional or prolonged labor; medications used such as anesthesia (halothane), magnesium sulfate, tocolytics (all cause uterine relaxation); prolonged third stage (>30 minutes); interventions such as use of vacuum or forceps, internal manipulation for retained fragments; inverted uterus. (*Debriefing:* This patient had pitocin, a prolonged labor with prolonged third stage >1 hour, a vacuum extraction for delivery, episiotomy with 4th-degree laceration.)
4. Perform an accurate postpartum assessment, including vital signs; fundal check for placement, firmness; lochia check (follow hospital protocol, but it may include to describe blood loss by counting/weighing pads and chux, recording the amount in specific time increments); perineal check(describe any signs of lacerations, hematoma, etc.—use REEDA scale).
5. Educate patient regarding her status, provide accurate information, offer an opportunity to ask questions, and let her know when to contact nurse (e.g., saturation of >1 pad in ≤1 hour). Also, educate patient on normal findings and have her palpate her uterus and recognize firmness.
6. Determine religious preference to establish if blood transfusions will be permitted (if they become necessary).
7. Given findings, evaluate more closely for hemorrhage:
   a. Monitor rate and quality of respirations.
   b. Measure pulse rate and quality (direct palpation) (increased 120 from 100).
   c. Compare blood pressure to baseline (dropped to 65/45 from 90/60).
   d. Inspect skin for pallor, coldness, clamminess, or cyanosis (pale, cool, clammy).
   e. Assess blood loss: lochia/clots, weight of pads, amount in given time.
   f. Evaluate level of consciousness.

The scenario also allows students to practice key elements from the National Council of State Boards of Nursing (NCSBN, 2007) National Council Licensure Examination for Registered Nurses (NCLEX-RN) test plan, including:

Safe and Effective Care Environment
    Management of Care
        Advocacy
        Collaboration With Interdisciplinary Team
        Establishing Priorities
    Safety and Infection Control
        Accident Prevention
        Error Prevention
Health Promotion and Maintenance
        Ante/Intra/Postpartum and Newborn Care
        Principles of Teaching/Learning
        Techniques of Physical Assessment
Psychosocial Integrity
        Crisis Intervention
        Religious and Spiritual Influences on Health
        Therapeutic Communications

Physiological Integrity
    Basic Care and Comfort
        Elimination
    Pharmacological and Parenteral Therapies
        Parenteral/Intravenous Therapies
        Pharmacological Agents/Actions
        Pharmacological Pain Management
    Reduction of Risk Potential
        Laboratory Values
        Potential for Alterations in Body Systems
        Potential for Complications From Surgical Procedures and Health
          Alterations
        System Specific Assessments
        Vital Signs
    Physiological Adaptation
        Hemodynamics
        Medical Emergencies
        Pathophysiology

For this scenario, the American Association of Colleges of Nursing (1998) *Essentials of Baccalaureate Education for Professional Nursing Practice* items addressed include the following:

■ Employ a range of technologies that facilitate patient care, including patient education and patient safety.
■ Integrate clinical data from all relevant sources of technology to inform the delivery of care.
■ Use professional communication and collaborative skills to deliver evidence-based, patient-centered care.
■ Demonstrate the application of psychomotor skills for the efficient, safe, and compassionate delivery of patient care.
■ Deliver appropriate patient-centered teaching that reflects developmental stage, age, culture, and health literacy considerations.
■ Implement holistic, patient-centered care that reflects an understanding of pathophysiology, pharmacology, medical management, and nursing management across the health-illness continuum (i.e., from primary care to home care to acute care to follow-up).
■ Implement evidence-based nursing interventions as appropriate for managing the acute and chronic care of patients and promoting health across the life span (e.g., acute and chronic pain, mobility, nutrition, skin care, oral, hydration, elimination, falls prevention, infection prevention, etc.).

Setting the Scene:

Equipment needed:

■ Medium-fidelity HPS on hospital bed
■ Video recording device (optional)
■ Projection screen (optional)

- Pulse oximeter
- Patient bracelet, with numbers to match to infant
- Gloves
- Intravenous setup (not connected), with these options for use: 1000 mL D5NS, Ringer, or normal saline)
- BP cuff and stethoscopes (alcohol wipes)
- Tubing and blood products
- Clean pads, gauze panties, pericare bottle

Resources needed:

- Medication record (see additional digital materials)
- Student activity checklist

Participant roles:

- Handler (person in control room or managing the medium-fidelity HPS) to change settings in response to student actions and speak for the patient in response to student questions
- Student to role-play the night nurse delivery report
- Faculty who serves as CNM on call for the patient during the day shift who can create orders and assist with care of patient

Scenario Implementation:

Initial Settings

- Apply wrist band.
- Have a printout of medications available to students on request.
- Simulate facial grimacing, diaphoresis on human HPS.
- Pad with large blood stain and two plum-size clots on HPS with gauze.
- Saline lock in with IV setup available.
- VS set at BP: 90/60, P: 100, RR: 16, T: 98.5 initially, with trend to change to BP: 65/45, P: 120, RR: 16, T: 101 over the first 5 minutes of students entering the room.

Required Student Assessments and Actions

- Reflect on patient risk status for PPH given past obstetric history and delivery history.
- Wash hands.
- Introduce self.
- Check name band.
- Assess general condition.
- Assess vital signs.
- Note difference from night report, rechecks BP and pulse.
- Apply pulse oximetry.
- Check capillary refill.
- Don gloves to do fundus, lochia, and perineal check.

- Ask patient when last urinated.
- Ask patient if passing gas (flatus).
- Note boggy fundus, large amount lochia with clots, and episiotomy with 4th-degree laceration 11/14 REEDA scale.
- Massage fundus.
- Apply pulse oximetry.
- Notice patient's complaints of pain and diaphoresis.
- Fundus remains boggy, bleeding continues.
- Call for help.
- Administer oxytocin 10 U IV through second setup placed in the lowest port.
- Re-evaluate fundus—it is firm.

Instructor Interventions

- Act as CNM and help students recognize obstetric medical emergency, direct their care.
- Debriefing of scenario.

Evaluation Criteria:

Checklist of Interventions and Assessments

_____ Wash hands.
_____ Introduce self.
_____ Check name band.
_____ Ask how patient is doing.
_____ Ask about pain level on 1 to 10 scale.
_____ Notice patient is sweating, cold, and clammy.
_____ Check hep-lock site for any signs of infections.
_____ Assess vital signs.
    _____ BP
    _____ P
    _____ RR
    _____ T
_____ Find abnormal P/BP/T.
_____ Recheck BP.
_____ Don gloves.
_____ Palpate fundus.
_____ Find fundus boggy and displaced to right.
_____ Ask if urinating.
_____ Ask last time up to urinate and amount urinated.
_____ Assess lochia.
_____ Find lochia bright red, heavy, with two plum-size clots.
_____ Maintain composure so as not to alarm patient.
_____ Massage fundus.
_____ Apply pulse oximetry.
_____ Assess further patient's complaints of pain—site and location—on a scale of 1 to 10.

_____ Find that fundus remains boggy, bleeding continues regardless of massage.

_____ Call for help.

_____ Report to CNM (by phone) what is going on.

_____ Determine need for oxytocic to contract uterus.

_____ Administer oxytocin 10 U IV.

_____ Determine need for pain medication.

_____ Administer Percocet 2 tabs po.

_____ Determine need for increased blood volume.

_____ Administer D5NS under CNM direction/order.

_____ Re-evaluate fundus.

_____ Find fundus firm.

_____ Set up plan for monitoring of high-risk patient (including getting infant in to breast-feed).

G. Debriefing Guidelines

Issues to consider:

- Patient history: Redhead, multiparity, large infant, difficult labor, medications, vacuum-assisted delivery, episiotomy with 4th-degree laceration.
- Infant not in to breast-feed since midnight (breast-feeding provides a natural oxytocic effect that can help decrease risk of PPH and excess bleeding).
- Potential bladder distention (given fundal right displacement above umbilicus).
- Episiotomy with 4th-degree laceration not checked since patient arrived from labor and delivery—risk of infection.
- Other signs and symptoms in patient that indicate potential for hemorrhage and shock: Change in vital signs (ˆpulse, decreasing BP), decreasing HgB and Hct from admission, patient's complaints of pain, patient diaphoresis.
- Conflicting issues: ROM >24 hours; vacuum aspiration (risk factors for infection); patient with fever, REEDA scale of 11/14 on 4th-degree laceration; questionable odor to lochia (all signs of infection).
- Outline other outcomes of this situation: If bleeding cannot be stopped, then surgery might be necessary and, ultimately, in the case of retained placenta or such situations, a hysterectomy may be performed. Helping the mother deal with the grief and outcome of this situation will be a challenge.

Student questions:

1. What challenges did you face?
2. What would you do differently next time?
3. Identify nursing diagnoses/problems for this patient (e.g., deficit fluid volume related to postpartum hemorrhage, anxiety related to sudden changes

in health status, risk for infection related to invasive procedures as a result of delivery and postpartum hemorrhage).

4. Outline a plan of care for this patient—identify specific nursing interventions for each area.

5. Is there other information you needed to adequately care for this patient (from report, lab values, etc.)?

6. How did you feel about caring for this otherwise young, healthy, vibrant woman who is suddenly in such apparent and life-threatening distress?

H. Suggestions/Key Features to Replicate or Improve

This scenario has been used very much "on the fly" without the carefully developed parameters that exist now. It will be used in this form in the next academic year with all of the new equipment and staff in place.

Some things that will be included, given others' experience:

- The use of a list of "student preparation" guidelines, including readings, videos, and other learning that will assist in their enactment of this experience.
- Enhancing the realism of the scenario by having Mrs. Jones answer student questions directly via microphone from the HPS.
- I envision that preparing the pad with its two plum-size clots will be a little messy.
- Having medications on hand for students to give in this type of "crisis" situation may be expecting too much given their past experience with simulations.
- This may be best used very near to the end of the semester, and as the course is now being taught over two semesters, the Fall first-semester senior nursing students should be more prepared to handle this high-risk medical obstetric emergency.

I. Recommendations for Further Use

This scenario is really a high-risk case that could be used to educate newly training staff to family birthing units and obstetric floors as well as undergraduate and graduate nursing students. In fact, the author is in contact with the manager of a family birthing unit at a local hospital to include new graduates this next academic year in the running of this scenario. FNP, WHNP, and CNM students would benefit from being part of this scenario. Late postpartum hemorrhage (after 24 hours) can happen after discharge from the hospital and might be detected in outpatient clinics by these practitioners. In addition, it could provide an opportunity for competency testing and accreditation checklists for hospitals that require a demonstration of staff's ability to manage obstetric emergencies.

J. Discussion of Simulation-Based Pedagogy and How This New Technology Has Contributed to Improved Student Outcomes

■ This scenario was developed to test the student's ability to perform an accurate postpartum assessment and take the actions necessary when abnormal results are found.

■ Having collaboration between faculty and lab staff for the actual running of the scenario is key.

■ Determine the best timing in the curriculum of the course and in the availability of the rooms and colleagues to assist.

■ Perform the scenario at the beginning of class to lead into the discussion of postpartum complications.

■ Integrate student in the classroom by assigning specific questions or jobs while the scenario is playing out.

■ During the debriefing, encourage the student who participated to provide some of their own feedback first to decrease their feelings of evaluation by others.

■ Focus on positive aspects of what students did well.

■ Gently introduce ideas about challenges or barriers to good care so that all students can participate in the brainstorming and critical thinking necessary to come up with new ideas.

■ Have student journal for a few minutes afterward to reflect on the experience. See if anyone is willing to share.

■ Have clinical faculty observe student postpartum assessments after the scenario and note any significant changes. Have the students reflect on this in their final journaling for the course.

References

American Association of Colleges of Nursing. (1998). *Essentials of baccalaureate education for professional nursing practice*. Washington, DC.: AACN.

Connecticut Health and Education Facilities Authority. (2007). CHEFA grant for $99,999.00, Women's Health Simulation Expansion. Project. Pilot Team: Suzanne Campbell (P.I.), Diana DeBartolomeo Mager (Co-P.I.), Phil Greiner, Sheila Grossman, and Alison Kris.

Davidson, M. R., London, M. L., & Ladewig, P. W. (2008), *Olds' maternal-newborn nursing & women's health across the lifespan* (8th ed., pp. 743–745, 1159–1165). Upper Saddle River, NJ: Pearson Prentice-Hall.

National Council of State Boards of Nursing. (2007). *NCLEX-RN examination: Test plan for the National Council Licensure Examination for Registered Nurses*. Retrieved June 18, 2008, from https://www.ncsbn.org/RN_Test_Plan_2007_Web.pdf

Recommended Readings

Bendetti, T. (2002). Obstetric hemorrhage. In S. Gabbe, J. Niebyl, & J. Simpson (Eds.), *Obstetrics: Normal and problem pregnancies* (4th ed.). New York: Churchill Livingstone.

Cunningham, F. G., Gant, N. F., Leveno, K. J., Gilstrap, L. C., III, Hauth, J. C., & Wenstrom, K. D. (2005). *Williams obstetrics* (22nd ed.). New York: McGraw-Hill.

Gilbert, E. S., & Harmon, J. S. (2003). *Manual of high risk pregnancy and delivery* (3rd ed.). St. Louis, MO: Mosby.

Gülmezoglu, A., Forna, F., Villar, J., & Hofmeyr, G. (2004). Prostaglandins for prevention of postpartum haemorrhage. In *The Cochrane Database of Systematic Reviews* (2006, Issue 3). Chichester, UK: John Wiley & Sons.

Lowdermilk, D. L., & Perry, S. E. (2007). *Maternity & women's health care* (9th ed.). St. Louis, MO: Mosby, Elsevier.

Magann, E., Evans, S., Chauhan, S., Lanneau, G., Fisk, A., & Morrison, J. (2005). The length of the third stage of labor and the risk of postpartum hemorrhage. *Obstetrics and Gynecology, 105*(2), 290–293.

MacMullen, N., Dulski, L., & Meagher, B. (2005). Red alert: Perinatal hemorrhage. *MCN American Journal of Maternal-Child Nursing, 30*(1), 46–51.

Poole, J. H., & White, D. (2005). *Obstetrical emergencies for the perinatal nurse* (2nd ed.). White Plains, NY: March of Dimes.

Roman, A. S., & Rebarber, A. (2003). Seven ways to control postpartum hemorrhage. *Contemporary OB/GYN, 48*(3), 34–36, 38, 41–42.

Shevell, T., & Malone, F. D. (2003). Management of obstetrical hemorrhage. *Seminars in Perinatology, 27*(1), 86–104.

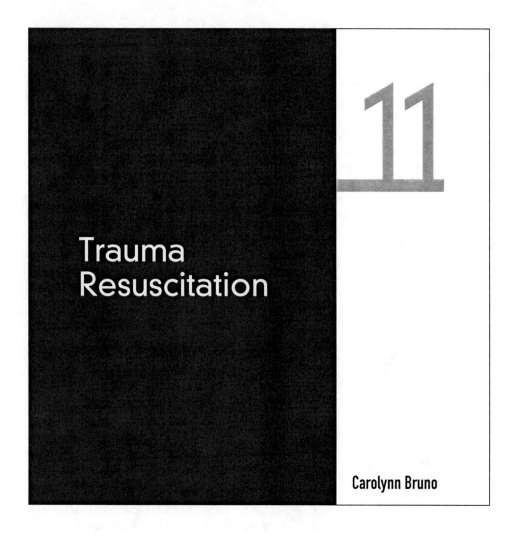

11

Trauma Resuscitation

Carolynn Bruno

A. Discussion of Implementation of Simulation-Based Pedagogy in Each Contributor's Individualized Teaching

Simulation-based learning occurs in an innovative fashion for baccalaureate nursing students at Western Connecticut State University (WCSU). Integrated simulation learning is utilized within the seminar portion of the critical care curriculum. It serves as an adjunct modality and is considered part of clinical time. The objective of simulation-based pedagogy in the curriculum is to provide an opportunity for baccalaureate students to acquire critical care skills that they may not otherwise encounter in the clinical setting. The application of high-fidelity simulation lends itself to providing safe practice that can occur in a nonthreatening environment with support from faculty and peers. Repetition to high-risk clinical situations desensitizes the anxiety component of students responding and participating in the delivery of high-acuity trauma resuscitation. Additionally, the students develop an "algorithm of response," learned behaviors of rapid assessment and nursing intervention, formulated on evidence-based practice that may be employed during any precode, code, or resuscitation occurrence.

B. Description of Educational Materials Available in Your Teaching Area and Relative to Your Specialty

Two of the three simulation facilities used at WCSU are designed to mirror critical care bays. These designated laboratories are available for nursing students to practice skills and enhance contextual learning. An additional ICU laboratory will be completed in the next fiscal year, supported by federal assistance. The ICU simulation facility that is used for the critical care course houses a hospital bed, ventilator, emergency equipment, and the human patient simulator (HPS) with remote PDA access. There are two adjoining laboratories, a classroom for instruction, and a smaller room designed as a library with textbooks. Computer access is available in the classroom with DVD/VHS and a large screen. The simulation room is of generous proportion, and there is space to divide the class reasonably and provide a quiet, private environment to run the simulation and debrief.

C. Specific Objective for Simulation Utilization Within a Specific Course and the Overall Program

The overall objective of integrating simulation within the framework of the course curriculum is to enhance student proficiency in performing critical care assessments and skills. Basic proficiency of appropriate nursing response to precode situations is imperative. Student nurses may have an opportunity to develop these skills with the assistance of simulation. This will alleviate anxiety and provide an arsenal of responsive techniques to employ when delivering care to critically ill patients. Role play and alternating these assignments facilitates teamwork and communication while providing safe care. An additional objective for student performance while working with high-fidelity simulation is to formulate pertinent differential diagnoses. While some would argue that this is not a function of the role of nursing or consistent with the students' novice level, it is critical to assist students to anticipate nursing interventions based on the patient's medical presentation. Providing case scenarios whereby students can process and synthesize medical diagnoses builds confidence and proficiency while delivering excellent nursing care.

D. Introduction of Scenario to Include Setting the Scene, Technology Used, Objectives, and Description of Participants

Students are introduced to the HPS with as much reality as possible. The sites, sounds, and smells of the trauma bay are difficult to replicate. One way to address this may be to play an audiotape of background sounds customarily heard during trauma resuscitation. For the purpose of this simulation, the patient is arrayed as a trauma patient would be. Access to all the medical equipment in the ICU lab is available. Technology available for use includes oxygen and emergency resuscitation equipment, stethoscopes, ventilator, cardiac monitor, hemodynamic monitoring lines, IVs and IV pump, code cart, NGT, suction equipment, Pleurovac drainage kit, and Foley catheter.

The objectives of the participants are as follows:

1. Recognize precode indicators leading to acute deterioration of trauma patient.
2. Perform basic trauma assessment.
3. Identify factors that place patient at risk for physiologic deterioration.
4. Increase proficiency in performing critical care skills.
5. Assume roles to enhance proficiency in the clinical area.
6. Communicate effectively within team framework.
7. Participate in debriefing exercise.
   a. Identify stressors.
   b. Identify areas for improvement (assessment, intervention, reevaluation, communication, team proficiency).

E. Describe Running of the Scenario

Students are introduced to assigned emergency department (ED) roles. They are offered a clipboard and record data on a mock critical care flow sheet and medication record. Professional observers would be assigned to record elapsed time and interventions. Data from the trauma scenario is introduced as a "call in" from the paramedic as the trauma patient is transported to the ED. The "nursing staff" has only minutes to set up emergency equipment necessary for the first few minutes of initial resuscitation. Written resource materials are not readily available apart from IV drip calculation sheets. Access to learning resources are kept minimal, as this is similar to that experienced in a live resuscitation.

The trauma patient is unmasked, and the resuscitation is in play. Students are expected to proceed using available technology resources and personnel. Trauma resuscitation knowledge is based on previous lecture content. The instructor provides patient data sequentially outlined in the scenario template. Coaching and cues are offered as the scenario unfolds. Typically, assistance in recognizing differential medical diagnoses is provided. Additional prompts include timeliness of interventions, recognition of elapsed time, and communication. Delegation is also a professional skill with which novice student nurses require additional assistance. Competency of skills seems sound overall. Positive reinforcement is consistently offered with the completion of appropriate assessments, recognition of differential diagnoses, successful nursing interventions, and effective communication.

F. Presentation of Completed Template

Twenty-four students divided into two groups were introduced to the assignment. Groups of 12 students were considered large. Several students were assigned roles as extra observers. Groups of six students would be ideal. To offset the large class size during simulation, three trauma simulations were run, and roles were rotated. Additional exercises aimed at identification of cardiac dysrhythmias, hemodynamic waveforms, and instability were offered within the scenario.

Title: Trauma Resuscitation
Clinical Nursing Practice III, Nursing 335 (Critical Care Curriculum)

Focus Area: ED Trauma Scenario for seniors and second-semester juniors

Scenario Description:

Client profile: Sally Snooze is a 21-year-old Caucasian college student brought into the ED on Friday night after crashing her Jeep Cherokee Sport Vehicle on I-84. EMTs report that Sally, the restrained driver, sustained anterior chest injuries. The airbag was deployed, and vomit was detected on the dashboard. Sally smelled of alcohol. At the scene, Sally was found alert but disoriented to place and short of breath, with acute chest pain 7/10 radiating to the thoracic area. Interventions at the scene include applying a cervical collar and backboard, O_2 at 4 L per minute, and a large bore peripheral IV of lactated Ringer at 125 cc per hour. The initial Glasgow coma scale indicates a score of 14, BP 90/60, P 126 beats per minute and irregular, and RR of 30 breaths per minute; respirations are shallow and decreased to the right mid and lower lobe. Sally is taken by ambulance to the ED trauma bay of a nearby Level I trauma center.

On arrival to the ED, paradoxical breathing and hemoptysis are present. Breath sounds are absent to the right midlobular region. It is determined that a chest tube should be placed to the right thorax. The chest tube immediately drains 200 cc of sanguinous fluid, and the Pleuravac is placed to 20 cm of suction. The patient is writhing on the hospital bed and moaning, "My chest hurts bad." Her level of consciousness (LOC) deteriorates, and she begins to vomit. A blood gas is drawn and demonstrates a PaO_2 of 86%. The patient is given IV sedation by the CRNA and is nasally intubated. Bibasilar breath sounds are present. A Swan Ganz catheter is placed to the left subclavian region with LR wide open and to monitor. BP is 84/50, P 144, and RR 12 breaths per minute and regular; O_2 sat is 98% on FiO_2 of 40%, AC-12, TV-800, no peep. The cardiac monitor shows sinus tachycardia with PVCs. JVD is present and is accompanied by muffled heart sounds. Faint peripheral pulses are palpable, and skin is cool and moist. A suprapubic abrasion with a red, 5 × 8 cm line of demarcation is noted. A nasogastric tube is inserted and placed at 60 cm continuous suction. A right radial arterial line is inserted by the CRNA. A 16 Fr. indwelling Foley catheter is placed to straight drainage with 200 cc of serosanguinous tinged urine output present. Soft wrist restraints are placed on the patient to avoid self-discontinuation of treatment modalities. An ABG, CBC with diff, chemistry panel, serum troponin, type and cross for 4 U, and blood alcohol level are drawn from the arterial line. An EKG reveals ST elevation in anterior leads. A C-spine radiograph and CXR are taken. The SG catheter and nasal endotracheal tube are confirmed to be properly placed on CXR. A resolving hemothorax to the right mid lobe is present on CXR. Focused Abdominal Sonography for Trauma (FAST) and an abdominal and pelvic U/S are ordered.

Past medical history (reported by patient's parents): S/P T & A at age 15 years; no chronic illnesses except for occasional UTIs

Family history: Lives with parents and two younger siblings, ages 19 and 15 years, all are A & W

Social History: College student majoring in criminal justice at a local university; employed in a work study program in the university library; "A" student; well liked by peers and has many friends, including a boyfriend whom she has dated exclusively for two years.

Psychiatric History: None

Immunizations: Up to date

Allergies: Morphine sulfate produces itching; PCN produces hives

Current medications: Multivitamin × 1 daily; oral contraceptive pill

Tobacco: None

Alcohol/Drugs: Drinks socially on weekends; no other substance usage known.

Scenario Objectives:

1. Maintains medical and surgical asepsis.
2. Performs basic trauma assessment.
3. Generates differential medical diagnoses pertinent to the initial assessment.
4. Identifies primary nursing interventions.
5. Recognizes factors that place patient at risk for physiologic deterioration.
6. Increases proficiency in critical care skills management.
7. Assumes roles to enhance proficiency and communication in trauma resuscitation.
8. Collaborates effectively with interdisciplinary team regarding crisis intervention.
9. Delegates nursing responsibilities to each team member.
10. Enacts emergency response plan.
11. Provides the need for interaction with family to maintain structural integrity.
12. Uses safety devices appropriately.
13. Participates in debriefing exercise.
    a. Identify stressors.
    b. Review areas for improvement (assessment, intervention, reevaluation, safety, communication, team proficiency).

All scenarios, National Council of State Boards of Nursing (NCSBN) RN test plan categories (NCSBN, 2007), addressed are as follows:

Safe and Effective Care Environment
Management of Care
Collaboration with Interdisciplinary Team
Consultation
Delegation
Establishing Priorities
Informed Consent
Referrals
Safety and Infection Control
Emergency Response Plan

Injury Prevention
Standard/Transmission-Based/Other Precautions
Safe Use of Equipment
Use of Restraints/Safety Devices
Health Promotion and Maintenance
Family Systems
High Risk Behaviors
Immunizations
Principles of Teaching/Learning
Techniques of Physical Assessment
Psychosocial Integrity
Chemical and Other Dependencies
Crisis Intervention
Grief and Loss
Unexpected Body Image Changes
Physiological Integrity
Basic Care and Comfort
Elimination
Mobility/Immobility
Pharmacological and Parenteral Therapies
Central Venous Access Devices
Parenteral/Intravenous Therapies
Reduction of Risk Potential
Diagnostic Tests
Laboratory Values
Potential for Alterations in Body Systems
Potential for Complication of Diagnostic Tests/Treatments/
Procedures
Potential for Complications from Surgical Procedures and Health
Alterations
System Specific Assessments
Therapeutic Procedures
Vital Signs
Physiological Adaptation
Alterations in Body Systems
Fluid and Electrolyte Imbalances
Hemodynamics
Illness Management
Medical Emergencies

Setting the Scene:

The scene was set in a designated critical care simulation room in a university setting. Federal assistance to expand the room capacity and technology will be appreciated in the next fiscal year. HPS on a hospital bed was utilized with cardiac monitor in place, ventilator support, NTT, Ambu bag, oxygen, code cart equipped with a defibrillator, central line catheters, IV machine with IV tubing, IV solution and meds, Pleuravac, NGT with suction canister, BP cuff, stethoscopes, automated BP cuff, and Foley catheters were available. Students are to record on trauma flow sheets and medication records. Interventions and time elapsed are recorded. The simulation level used high fidelity during the trauma scenario. Remote PDA access was available. Students had access to a substantial 17″ screen to visualize the cardiac rhythm, hemodynamic profile including CVP and PA readings, and arterial waveforms.

Groups of 12 students each participated in HPS case scenarios. Each student nurse assumed assigned roles, including two trauma team responders, three ED nursing staff, one recorder, two runners, and four observers. Written scripts were not observed but would be useful in future simulation exercises. Students had nearby access to text resources, medication books, references, and laptops. The exercise, however, was to mimic a real-life trauma resuscitation scenario, so the use of resources during the resuscitation phase were minimal by design.

Three trauma scenarios were executed in approximately 45 minutes. Debriefing accounted for 15 minutes additional time per scenario run. Informal scripts were verbally provided for each player in the scene. Several students played the role of professional observer and were helpful in providing the response team with differential diagnoses, verbalizing appropriate nursing interventions, and keeping track of time elapsed.

Scenario Implementation:

Initial Settings for the Human Patient Simulator
BP: 90/60, P: 126 beats per minute and irregular, RR: 30 breaths per minute.

Required Student Action and Interventions

- Focused trauma assessment and alcohol evaluation.
- Identify need to place chest tube and assists in chest tube insertion following protocol for insertion, assessment, and care.
- Continue frequent respiratory assessment.
- Focused cardiac assessment with recommendations for interventions.
- NGT placement and assessment of proper placement.
- IV access obtained.
- Foley catheter insertion.
- Identify blood tests.

____ Draw labs and sends for the following tests (ABG, CBC with diff, chemistry panel, serum troponin, type and cross for 4 U, blood alcohol level).

Instructor Interventions
Students have required some cues with basic communication skills. Asking "who is in charge?" helps them get started with communication and delegation skills. Asking the professional observer to provide a time check and summarizing the various assessments and interventions that have been performed helps to keep on track. Occasional attention to hemodynamic waveforms is requested. Clinical prompts to note respiratory pattern, muffled heart sounds, and safety measures in the form of soft wrist restraints may be necessary. The ventilator is an unfamiliar piece of equipment. Prompts to interface with it are made.

Evaluative Criteria:

This scenario was implemented without specific criteria to rate individual competency in performing skills during resuscitation. Students came to the scenario with competencies previously measured in another course. The simulation exercise involved group participation. It would be further enhanced in the future with specific criteria to measure individual competencies performed. Additional instructor support would be necessary.

Students will be evaluated based on the degree to which he or she performs the skill in the appropriate order. Attention to the need for prompts are considered (see Table 11.1).

G. Debriefing Guidelines

At the conclusion of the trauma scenario, the simulation was discontinued and 15 minutes were allowed for debriefing and evaluation. The team's effort as it related to trauma care, communication, delegation, appropriateness, and timeliness of interventions and the attentiveness to family needs were reviewed. Questions and points to review posed to the group were as follows:

1. What were the identified risk factors present in this case scenario?
2. Review the components of the primary assessment and secondary survey. Were the assessments complete? Did these assessments progress in a proper and timely sequence? If not, what were the factors that impeded the progression of the surveys?
3. What were the indicators of deterioration in the patient's condition?
4. List applicable differential diagnoses.
5. Based on the differential diagnosis list, which were the priority nursing interventions? Were these offered? If so, were these executed in a timely fashion?
6. Was written documentation maintained properly?
7. Was communication among team members clear?
8. Were roles clearly defined? Was there overlap? If so, was the overlap helpful or prohibitive?
9. Were proper referrals to the interdisciplinary team members made in a timely fashion?
10. Which referrals were made?
11. Was the patient's family/significant others cared for? Where were they placed during the resuscitation? Which members of the interdisciplinary team stayed with them to answer questions and offer support? When were they allowed to see the patient?
12. Did the scenario proceed in a timely and realistic fashion?
13. What overall improvements would you make when running this scenario again?
14. Which stressors have you identified?
15. Did you find the scenario was beneficial to your learning about trauma care? Explain.

11.1 Evaluating Student Criteria in a Nursing Simulation Scenario

Behavior	Independent	Prompting	Appropriate Order
Maintain medical and surgical asepsis			
Perform basic trauma assessment			
Generate differential medical diagnoses pertinent to initial assessment			
Identify primary nursing interventions			
Recognize factors that place patient at risk for physiologic deterioration			
Increase proficiency in critical care skills management			
Assume roles to enhance proficiency and communication in trauma resuscitation			
Collaborate effectively with interdisciplinary team regarding crisis intervention			
Delegate nursing responsibilities to each team member			
Enact emergency response plan			
Provide the need for interaction with family to maintain structural integrity			
Use safety devices appropriately			
Participate in debriefing exercises			
Identify stressors			
Review areas for improvement: assessment, intervention, reevaluation, safety, communication, and team proficiency			

H. Suggestions/Key Features to Replicate or Improve

Suggestions to facilitate new learning would be to keep interventions simple. Allow students to formulate nursing interventions based on the top three medical differential diagnoses. In this trauma scenario, the priority nursing diagnoses were ineffective breathing pattern, risk for aspiration and decreased cardiac output related to cardiac tamponade, dysrhythmia, and/or shock secondary to organ trauma. Allow students to rerun the scenario after debriefing to integrate newly acquired knowledge and skills.

Additions to improve the simulation would include an audiotape of ED sounds to introduce the students to the potential distractions during the exercise. The ability for students to remain focused on the task and to delimit peripheral distraction would improve their delivery of care. The provision of a formalized checklist of skills performed would be helpful. Also, delimiting the group to a size of six students would be ideal. Individualized evaluation would be made easier. The aim of this scenario was mainly group process and teamwork. Having additional instructors present to record individual performance would add dimension to this exercise.

I. Recommendations for Further Use

During the running of this simulation, I would recommend that the patient condition does not resolve completely after each successful intervention. Although this would prove extraordinary, it does not reflect the reality of resuscitation. It risks limiting the scope of critical thinking and group process that one hopes to achieve through the exercise. The inclusion of some student-generated deviations was also allowed during the scenario. This proved to add great fun to the debriefing component of the exercise.

The trauma scenario would be recommended for use in critical care courses, competency review and evaluation for nurses new to critical care, mock code training, acute-care nurse practitioner education, and medical school education.

J. Discussion of Simulation-Based Pedagogy and How This New Technology Has Contributed to Improved Student Outcomes

Simulation-based pedagogy is a unique and creative adjunct that adds dimension to nursing education. It provides opportunity for adaptive learning in a proactive, linear fashion. Acquired skills and competencies are fused in a safe, contextual manner during simulation exercises. A simulation scenario provides exposure to high-acuity skills the student might not otherwise master as a novice nurse. Application of advanced critical thinking skills occurs in live time with instantaneous measurable outcomes. The student has an opportunity to develop a set of algorithms for responsive behaviors in a supportive environment. These approaches are accomplished while alleviating student anxiety that normally accompanies a live patient encounter. The mastery of critical care skills is consolidated within the construct of the nursing process: assessment, nursing diagnosis, planning, intervention, and evaluation.

Simulation affords a safe environment for proactive learning that differs from traditional clinical encounters. Often, traditional learning occurs in a retrograde fashion. Students provide care for patients, and then after a period of reflection and integration, the nursing process is applied to the experience. In this manner, patient goals, interventions, and outcomes are measured and enhanced retrospectively. In simulation, instant recall of learned knowledge stored in the students' mental warehouse must be downloaded as the scenario rolls. The students evaluate the efficacy of their nursing interventions through immediate high-fidelity feedback. This feedback loop regulates self-correction with minimal instructor prompts. The instructor's role within the scenario is to coach. Intrinsically, learning is safe, adaptive, and fun. Student anxiety is lessened through repetitive practice of responsive actions. Debriefing as a group process provides insight into the broad strokes of applied knowledge and team effort.

References

National Council of State Boards of Nursing. (2007). *NCLEX-RN examination: Test plan for the National Council Licensure Examination for Registered Nurses*. Retrieved June 18, 2008, from https://www.ncsbn.org/RN_Test_Plan_2007_Web.pdf

Recommended Texts

Aehlert, B. (2003). *ECG's made easy 2E with companion evolve* (3rd ed.). St. Louis, MO: Mosby.

Smeltzer, S., Bare, B., Hinkle, J., & Cheever, K. (2008). *Brunner and Suddarth's textbook of medical-surgical nursing* (11th ed.). Philadelphia, PA: Lippincott.

Sole, M., Klein, D., & Moseley, M. (2005). *Introduction to critical care nursing* (4th ed.). St. Louis, MO: Elsevier.

12

Posttraumatic Stress Disorder/ Traumatic Brain Injury and Other Conditions in an Iraqi Veteran of War

Doris Troth Lippman

A. Discussion of Implementation of Simulation-Based Pedagogy in Each Contributor's Individualized Teaching

In my past 25 years of teaching both undergraduate and graduate psychiatric mental health nursing, I have used many forms of innovative teaching, including case studies, role-play, and clips from movies and DVDs, but simulation is new and in the early stages of development for this clinical specialty. I have a particular expertise in this area as a result of my service as a captain in the Army Nurse Corps during the conflict in Vietnam. I was stationed at the Seventh Field Hospital, where soldiers with traumatic wounds involving flesh and bones were sent to be treated. Their injuries were often so severe that they were unable to make it safely back home. After I returned to the United States in 1969, a time when the country was quite divided about the war, I did not revisit my Vietnam experience until 1980, when I took a group of junior nursing students for the psychiatric clinical experience to the West Haven VA in Connecticut. What struck me the most was the degree of emotional injury that existed in these soldiers who had returned from Vietnam years ago. It was not until 1980 that the *Diagnostic and Statistical Manual of Mental Disorders* (DSM-III) legitimized the condition as Post Traumatic Stress Disorder (PTSD). This condition develops as a result of being placed in a life-threatening position or being exposed to seeing others who are also so threatened. New onset, self-reported PTSD symptoms, or diagnosis among deployed military personnel with combat exposure occurred at about a threefold higher rate than in nondeployed military personnel according to Romo (2008).

B. Description of Educational Materials Available in Your Teaching Area and Relative to Your Specialty

At Fairfield University, the School of Nursing's Robin Kanarek Learning Resource Center was developed in 2006 and includes areas for high-fidelity manikin simulation as well as home health/psychiatric simulation. It is feasible to do a live interview in the simulation room (set up with couch and chairs) and video-feed live to a classroom where students could observe the interaction and individual or group therapy. We are experimenting with implementing a variety of strategies that can simulate actual nurse–patient interactions for student learning. The ideal for this simulation would be to have students conduct the interview with an actor playing the role of a veteran who had returned from Iraq/Afghanistan, and other students could observe the interview.

C. Specific Objective for Simulation Utilization Within a Specific Course and the Overall Program

The overall objectives of this scenario are to have the student conduct a mental status exam and a suicide assessment and evaluate economic, psychosocial, and other concerns of the client. However, what is particularly distressing to the student is that he or she knows that the suicide rate in Iraqi and Afghan veterans continues to increase each year and sometimes exceeds combat-related deaths of the conflict. Soldiers are committing suicide not only both in Iraq and Afghanistan but also when they come home. The rates this year, 2008, are already higher than those from 2007. These suicides include not only the men but also the women.

The women face an even greater service stress-related condition—being sexually abused and/or harassed by fellow soldiers. Oftentimes, this harassment is from unit members. This trauma has resulted in some instances of high levels of PTSD in the military. The military has tried to remedy these situations, but in many others, it is the military bureaucratic system that does not allow junior officers to report the behavior of their senior officers. Such behavior could result in court marshal and dishonorable discharge. Many military women are therefore trapped in a venue of silence. At the undergraduate level, students should recognize the need for an additional neurology consult for this patient. At the graduate level, it would be expected that students would recognize the need and administer the Acute Concussion Evaluation (ACE) tool to determine whether the soldier is suffering from traumatic brain injury (TBI) and to what degree. TBI is sudden physical damage to the brain. Closed head injuries, which are what soldiers in combat are often suffering from, can cause diffuse damage to several areas of the brain. The impact of the injury causes the brain to move back and forth against the inside of the bony skull. The major areas of the brain that are affected cause communication difficulties. Other problems may include swallowing, walking, and balance as well as changes in memory and cognitive skills. This simulation can be used in the mental health course as well as physiology/pharmacology/health assessment at both the undergraduate and graduate levels.

D. Introduction of Scenario to Include Setting the Scene, Technology Used, Objectives, and Description of Participants

The scene takes place in the office of a VA hospital APRN. A fellow Iraqi vet called the West Haven VA mental health line because he was concerned about his buddy who he had served with recently in Iraq. The patient and his buddy can either be volunteers (student, faculty member, lab director) or a high-fidelity human patient simulator (HPS) sitting in a wheelchair. If using high-fidelity HPS, the HPS can be a right-legged amputee at the knee. The person running the scenario can answer the questions via the HPS. If a volunteer is used, the scenario can be run with very little technology.

By the end of this session, the students will be able to do the following:

1. Conduct a suicide assessment
2. Perform a mental status exam
3. Recognize the economic, psychosocial, neurologic, and behavioral issues for veterans from WWII through Iraq and Afghanistan
4. Describe the different symptoms in PTSD Clusters (Intrusive, Avoidant, and Arousal)
5. Provide veteran with resource information (such as vet centers) to help with coming home issues
6. Ask client about exposure to explosive devices such as improvised explosive devices, roadside bombs, and land minds

E. Describe Running of the Scenario

The student will ask pertinent questions of the Iraqi veteran related to activities of daily living, mental status, social relationships, and present physical/mental/emotional health. The student observes the veteran's affect, manner, response to questions, and physical appearance and uses this information to guide further questions and specific evaluation using assessment tools. The person role-playing the Iraqi veteran should portray suicidal ideation, PTSD, TBI symptoms, and issues of self-esteem related to this multifaceted condition. The buddy should portray concern for his friend, honest evaluation of his friend's condition (e.g., TBI symptoms), and support.

F. Presentation of Completed Template

Title: PTSD/TBI and Other Conditions in an Iraqi Veteran of War

Focus Area: Mental health course, first-semester junior year BSN or first-semester freshman year ADN

Scenario Description:
Scenario Background History and Dialogue

(*Note:* Because of the psychiatric mental health focus of this simulation, the background history and dialogue is much more critical and needs to be much more in-depth.)

The returning soldier is 23 years old. He signed up for the Reserves to do his patriotic duty. He had no idea that he would be deployed to Iraq. He tells the student that he was only supposed to be in the country for 15 months, but his deployment kept being extended, which was very upsetting to him—"I never knew when I was going to get out of there!" He also shared with the nursing student that he saw many dead bodies, was fired at by the enemy, and saw many injured women and children. He also killed at least one of the enemy soldiers. He feels a great deal of guilt because he survived and many of his fellow soldiers did not.

He told the student that he knew from the news and newspapers that many soldiers had killed themselves or others and that he was having a lot of disturbing thoughts himself. When the student asked more specifically about what he was feeling, he mentioned nightmares, hypervigilance, and intrusive thoughts. The student noticed that even though he said "I feel fine," he had tears streaming down his face. He also shared that he was witness to many women both civilian and military being raped, and he felt he could not help for risk of being court marshaled and or dishonorably discharged.

He has been home for a month, and his wife just told him she is going to divorce him. He has been unable to find a job even though his previous employer promised to save it for him. Some of the other things he notices are that he often has trouble controlling his anger and finds himself engaging in road rage and other risky behaviors. When the student asks if he has thoughts of hurting himself, he responds "sometimes," but indicates when asked about a plan, he does not have one but does have access to a loaded weapon.

Student asks the veteran about any loss of consciousness that he might have had that lasted between a few seconds to 2 to 3 minutes In addition, questions about exposure to explosions are essential. Both of these have been linked to TBI. The soldier indicated that he had been exposed to multiple explosions when improvised explosive devices (IEDs) and other explosive devices were detonated. He remembers being told that he had lost consciousness on numerous occasions but has no memory of these events. He does, however, display classic symptoms of TBI such as inability to think and to remember or plan clearly enough to deal with the activities necessary for everyday living. The client also indicates that he has noticed some memory, vision, and hearing problems. He does indicate that the symptoms are mild, but the student knows that TBI injuries can accumulate over time, leading to serious neurologic problems. According to the neurologist evaluating his head x-rays, the blast under his Humvee caused enough damage so that his brain looked like Play-Doh®. (Berger, 2008).

The student asks the client about his ability to plan for daily activities. The vet looks at his buddy with a puzzled look. The buddy indicated that his friend had a great deal of difficulty with activities of daily living. The student does conduct a Mini Mental State Exam and finds symptoms that meet the criteria for PTSD on Axis I; Axis II is deferred; Axis III, amputation below right knee; Axis IV, problems with occupation and social relationships; and Axis V, global assessment of functioning (GAF), currently 50–60/100. She also conducts an ACE test to determine the presence and/or degree of TBI.

The nursing student had checked with her instructor before meeting with the client about possible referral information. The instructor suggested that the client be encouraged to continue to see his therapist and take medications that have been prescribed for him. The instructor, being a veteran herself, was aware of "Vet Centers" (http://www1.va.gov/directory/guide/vetcenter_flsh.asp?isFlash=1), which were established in 1979 to meet the readjustment needs of Vietnam veterans. Now, they are available for all veterans. She had the student encourage him to take advantage of these excellent resource centers.

Scenario Objectives:

1. Conduct a suicide assessment.
2. Perform a mini mental state exam.
3. Recognize the economic, psychosocial, neurologic, and behavioral issues for veterans from WWII through Iraq and Afghanistan.
4. Describe the different symptoms in PTSD Clusters (Intrusive, Avoidant, and Arousal).
5. Provide veteran with resource information (such as vet centers) to help with coming home issues.
6. Ask client about exposure to explosive devices such as IEDS, roadside bombs, and land mines.

The National Council Licensure Examination for Registered Nurses (NCLEX-RN) test plan categories and subcategories (NCSBN, 2007) addressed in this simulation include the following:

Safe and Effective Care Environment
  Management and Care
      Case Management
      Consultation
      Establishing Priorities
      Referrals
      Resource Management
  Safety and Infection Control
      Home Safety
  Health Promotion and Maintenance
      Expected Body Image Changes

High-risk Behaviors
Self-care Psychosocial Integrity
Crisis Intervention
Family Dynamics
Grief and Loss
Mental Health Concepts
Sensory/Perceptual Alterations
Situational Role Changes
Stress Management
Support Systems
Therapeutic Communication
Unexpected Body Image Changes
Physiological Integrity
Physiological Integrity
Reduction of Risk Potential
System Specific Assessments

Setting the Scene:

The scene takes place in the office of a VA hospital APRN. A fellow Iraqi vet called the West Haven VA mental health line because he was concerned about his buddy who he had served with recently in Iraq. The patient and his buddy are present, and the veteran is sitting in a wheelchair with a right leg amputation at the knee. The person running the scenario can answer the questions via the HPS. If a volunteer is used, the scenario can be run with very little technology.

Resources needed: Information about PTSD, TBI, sexual military trauma, access to assessment tools (Mini Mental Exam, ACE, PTSD, and suicide), textbooks, and computer access for database search and evidence-based practice.

Students need to prepare by reading up on the major areas outlined in this chapter and knowing how to perform the following assessments: mini mental exam and suicide for undergraduates with knowledge of some of the symptoms of PTSD. Use of the ACE assessment tool would be more appropriate for graduate-level students.

Faculty instructions for preparation: Same as above.

Simulator level: Live actors (veterans, retired professionals, acting students) preferred; high-fidelity HPS with the ability for immediate responses via microphone would be feasible

Participants needed:

Student as the nurse

Iraqi veteran (male); could also use a female Iraqi veteran who could address military sexual trauma experience

Buddy of vet

(See scenario description for script information.)

Scenario Implementation: Volunteer "vet" or HPS: right knee amputation, dressed in fatigues, wheelchair, office furniture with two chairs

Equipment needed:

- Volunteer or HPS seated in a wheelchair with fatigues on. He is wheeled in by one of his Army buddies, as his right leg was amputated below the knee by a mine that one of his fellow platoon members stepped on.
- Student to interview returning soldier sitting in a chair across from him.
- Approximately 30 minutes of time for the interview.

Instructor interventions: The instructor will enact one of two roles: if a volunteer is not available, instructor will "play" the veteran by use of the microphone to HPS; otherwise, if volunteer to role-play is present, instructor will be available in the room (with patient's permission) and assist the student with questioning as needed. Alternately, instructor could be outside the room, and after part of the interview, student could come with some questions for guidance (suggest use of assessment tools, veteran center referrals, etc.).

Evaluative Criteria: Students will be given feedback based on the degree to which they, in the appropriate order and with or without coaching, perform the actions (Table 12.1).

G. Debriefing Guidelines

Instructor may debrief with the student individually or may use several smaller groups of students. A summary of the debriefing outcomes might be helpful to share with all students.

Questions used for the debriefing:

1. How did you plan/prepare for your visit? Are any members of your family veterans? Do you know anyone who is currently serving in Iraq/Afghanistan?
2. What resources did you use to gather information?
3. What did you think when you walked in the room and saw the young amputee in his fatigues and in a wheelchair?
4. Have you ever cared for someone who has had an amputation? What physical and psychosocial issues might you need to include in his care?
5. What did you teach, and what else could you have taught the patient?
6. Do you think that with the patient's permission it would have been helpful to invite the person who brought him to the VA to come into the interview?
7. How does the terminology used affect the interaction/communication (e.g., better to use the word concussion instead of "mild traumatic brain injury" to increase communication)?
8. How did you feel when the veteran mentioned having a loaded gun at home?

H. Suggestions/Key Features to Replicate or Improve

The key concepts here are completing a mini mental health exam and a suicide assessment. Although the setting is at the primary care clinic at the veterans' hospital, it can also take place at a veterans center or another outpatient clinic.

12.1 Evaluating Student Criteria in a Nursing Simulation Scenario			
Behavior	Independent	Prompting	Appropriate Order/Comments
Introduce self to client			
Ask pertinent questions			
Properly wash hands			
Conduct a mental health assessment			
Conduct a suicide assessment			
Use proper interpersonal relations			
Ask about economic needs			
Ask about housing and other psychosocial needs			
Ask about TBI symptoms			
Refer for a neurologic workup			
Answer questions			
Say good-bye to patient			
Document			

TBI, traumatic brain injury.

I. Recommendations for Further Use

Since many veterans, especially those who have served in Vietnam, still have opinions related to coming home and the perception that the government did not do all it could to help them, I would recommend that the interviews not be conducted in a VA hospital but rather in another setting such as those mentioned previously.

References

Berger, D. (2008, May 25). The Sargeant [lost]. *New York Times Magazine,* 41–45.

National Council of State Boards of Nursing. (2007). *NCLEX-RN examination: Test plan for the National Council Licensure Examination for Registered Nurses.* Retrieved June 18, 2008, from https://www.ncsbn.org/RN_Test_Plan_2007_Web.pdf

Romo, J. M. (2008). *Combat veterans and post traumatic stress disorder.* Presentation at Lowell, Massachusetts, Vet Center, January 7, 2008.

Recommended Readings

Bolvin, J. (2008). Tales from Tikrit. *Nursing Spectrum Northeast, 12*(2), 22–23.

Fischer, C., & Reiss, D. (2006). The battle at home. *Registered Nurse: Journal of Patient Advocacy, 102*(8), 14–21.

Hoge, C. W., & Castro, C. A. (2004). Combat duty in Iraq and Afghanistan, mental health problems, and barriers to care. *New England Journal of Medicine, 351*(1), 13–22.

Hoge, C. W., McGurk, D., Thomas, J. L., Cox, A. L., Engel, C. C., & Castro, C. A. (2008). Mild traumatic brain injury in U.S. soldiers returning from Iraq. *New England Journal of Medicine, 358*(5), 453–463.

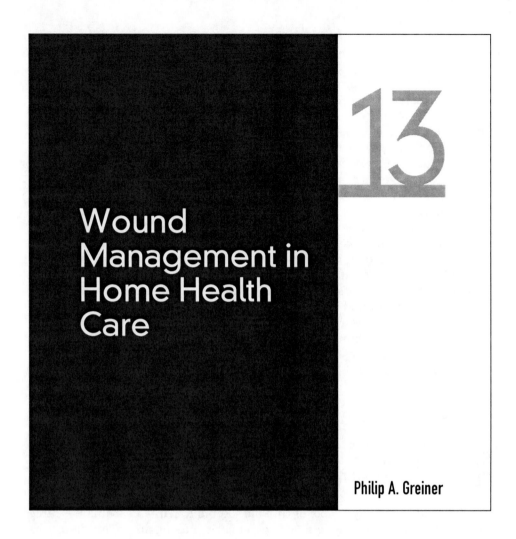

13

Wound Management in Home Health Care

Philip A. Greiner

A. Discussion of Implementation of Simulation-Based Pedagogy in Each Contributor's Individualized Teaching

Simulation has been used in the content area of public health and home health nursing for several years. From tabletop exercises in emergency preparedness to case studies in the classroom, simulation without manikins, with a single manikin, or with multiple manikins are all possible. Classroom use of case studies and role-play help students to understand situations that they are likely to encounter on home visits. The following scenario can be set up as a case study, a role-play and can use a static or high-fidelity human patient simulator (HPS) as the patient. In addition, a caregiver can be added by using another student, faculty, or actor in this role.

One of the most common problems addressed by nurses in home health care is management of wound care. With cost of hospitalization linked directly to length of stay, patients with wounds are discharged to home care as soon as possible after surgery. Added to this group of patients are those who developed wounds while hospitalized due to care deficits and/or secondary problems related to mobility, nutrition, or falls.

This chapter will address the critical components of a home health visit to a patient with a leg wound. The student will need to communicate with the patient and/or family member, assess the wound including current measurements and observations, decide on a course of action, and redress the wound. Documentation of the care provided is included in the scenario. Additional components may be added to this scenario to address common problems. For example, the patient or caregiver may have hearing loss or visual impairment.

Home management of wounds is different than in-hospital management on several levels. First, the patient and family are directly confronted with the costs associated with wound care. Charges for all dressings used are paid out of pocket and then submitted for reimbursement—if the patient has insurance coverage for these items. Second, wound care at home is done using clean technique. Without the risk of hospital-acquired infection, sterile technique becomes less important. Also, it simplifies the teaching required and skills necessary for family members to do wound redressings.

Simulations provide a method of teaching students, practicing home health nurses, and family members the skills and process components while allowing for mistakes. Simulations, and the DVD recordings of simulation sessions, are a new resource for nurses in this practice area. As more home care agencies adopt electronic medical record systems and nurses are equipped with laptop computers, DVDs of specific skills may provide a method of initial teaching before asking family members to actually perform the skill on a family member.

B. Description of Educational Materials Available in Your Teaching Area and Relative to Your Specialty

The Fairfield University School of Nursing's Robin Kanarek Learning Resource Center has a dedicated home health/psychiatric nursing area. This area, part of a larger room that houses the new maternal/newborn simulation area, is partitioned off from the larger area with storage units to form a small simulated bedroom. The area contains furniture donated by faculty members to create a typical bedroom in a low- to moderate-income home, complete with a single bed, nightstand, single chair with arms, and a bedside commode in a 12 × 8 ft. area. Either a low- or high-fidelity HPS may be used, or an actor may play the role of the patient.

For this scenario, the left leg is painted with washable paint to mimic a 4 cm × 3 cm wound. One section of the wound is painted with yellow-green paint to indicate an area of possible infection. The dressing covering the wound is a combination of 4 × 4s, an ABD dressing, and Kling wrap. No tape is used, except to secure the Kling wrap to itself—not to the manikin. The first 4 × 4 has green-tinted cream of wheat located on top of the green painted area of the wound. The room can be set up with trip hazards, such as lamp cords across the bedside area and a throw rug on the floor beside the bed.

The primary objective of this scenario is accurate assessment, appropriate wound care treatment, and documentation of the wound in a home health setting. Additional components may be added to address communication skills (with patient, family, supervisor, faculty, or primary care provider), completion of the OASIS database assessment, or supervision of a home health aide. The scenario is part of a final semester, fourth-year public health nursing course in a baccalaureate nursing program. Students in this semester have had theory and clinical courses in core health promotion, geriatric nursing, and basic medical nursing as well as all the specialty courses including mental health, acute medical-surgical, women's health and obstetrical, and pediatric nursing. As a result, students can be expected to understand the diagnoses, assessment, and management of chronic diseases, the care needs of older adults, and the appropriate use of medical therapeutics. Students in the public health nursing course have already had content on home and community assessment, the ecological model applied to health, and an asset-based approach to public health nursing.

The student will need an orientation to the patient similar to what might be expected from a primary nurse in the home care agency. A basic chart and summary of the last home health visit as well as a nursing bag may be added to increase realism.

C. Specific Objective for Simulation Utilization Within a Specific Course and the Overall Program

The objectives of this simulation are to determine the student's ability to do the following:

- Assess wound healing and the presence of infection.
- Correctly report findings to the most appropriate supervisory person.
- Communicate effectively with the patient, caregiver, primary nurse, faculty member, and physician.

This scenario can be used as the beginning activity for either class or clinical as part of the home care component of a public health nursing course or a medical-surgical nursing course. The students should have had skills content and theory related to home health care. Content on the conduct of a home visit and working with family caregivers is also important to include before conducting this scenario. The scenario should be recorded and reviewed as part of the debriefing process with the students involved. Particular attention should be paid to the reaction of the student to the signs of infection and the student's conveying of this information to the patient, caregiver, primary nurse, and faculty member. Documentation of the assessment, diagnosis, and care provided should be equally emphasized.

D. Introduction of Scenario to Include Setting the Scene, Technology Used, Objectives, and Description of Participants

Setting the Scene:
The students should be introduced to the scenario before entering the simulation room. The setting of the scenario is the patient's home.

It is important to set the scene by acting as if the transmission of the case information is taking place at the home health agency and the primary nurse is conveying the case information. The patient can be communicative by using a HPS or an actor, or the patient can be silent by using a low-fidelity HPS. If the patient is to be silent, a family caregiver (actor) should be present.

Technology Used
Technology used may vary in this scenario, depending on equipment available and the specific goal of the scenario. It may also be varied so that groups of student do not know what to expect.

Objectives
The National Council Licensure Examination for a Registered Nurse (NCLEX-RN) test plan categories and subcategories (NCSBN, 2007) addressed in the simulation include the following:

Safe and Effective Care Environment
> *Management of Care*
>> Client Rights
>> Concepts of Management
>> Establishing Priorities
> *Safety and Infection Control*
>> Handling Hazardous and Infectious Materials
>> Reporting of Incident/Event/Irregular Occurrence/Variance
>> Standard/Transmission-Based/Other Precautions

Health Promotion and Maintenance
>> Aging Process
>> Techniques of Physical Assessment

Physiological Integrity
> *Physiological Adaptation*
>> Alterations in Body Systems
>> Infectious Diseases

Description of Participants

Students: Student should be at the senior level, with sufficient content in nursing to make accurate assessments in the home. Student should be able to manage medically complex patients.

Patient: The patient is an older adult in a home setting. The scenario can be arranged to best represent the type of patient seen in local home health agencies. The amount of information that the patient shares with the student can vary depending on the additional objectives of the scenario.

Instructor: The instructor running the scenario should allow the students to decide on their approach to the patient, the assessment components necessary to provide care, the process of wound assessment, and the plan of action after determining that the wound is infected. The instructor may act as a resource for additional information but should allow the students to make all decisions.

E. Describe Running of the Scenario

This scenario will take place in a patient's home. The nursing students are assigned to make a home visit to the patient to assess cardiovascular status, assess the wound, and redress the wound using a dry, sterile dressing. Documentation and reporting is a key component of this scenario.

Student Preparation
Students should be in their final year of nursing education, with sufficient classroom and clinical experience to understand the basics of nutrition, movement, morbidities, and attitude on the development of wounds of the skin. Students will benefit from reading the references prior to the actual scenario. If mulage is used, be sure to warn students about eating well before the simulation is run. It is assumed that no food or drink is allowed in the simulation area.

F. Presentation of Completed Template

Title: Wound Management in Home Health Care

Focus Area:
Community Health, Health Assessment, Medical-Surgical Nursing

Scenario Description:
The patient is a 70-year-old black female living alone in a senior housing high-rise facility. She has a 15-year history of type II diabetes and an 18-year history of poorly controlled hypertension. These chronic conditions contributed to her development of peripheral vascular disease (PVD). She developed an ulcer on the lateral aspect of the left foot, measuring 3 cm × 2 cm (length by width) and 0.5 cm deep. She is unable to redress the wound herself and has no one available to do this for her. On this visit, the wound redressing is the priority.

One or two students should be assigned to "make the home visit." The students should introduce themselves, explain the purpose of the visit, ask permission to assess the wound, and proceed to do the wound assessment. As the dressing is removed, the students see a wound in the beginning stages of infection, with reddened areas around the edges and drainage (greenish-yellow) on the dressing. If video recording the scenario, try to capture the student's reaction to the appearance of the wound. The point of this scenario is to have the students decide next steps. The students should, or should be prompted to, explain to the patient what was found, contact the primary nurse or instructor to report the change in the wound, contact the primary care provider to report the change, and document the change accurately. The students should also finish redressing the wound.

Evaluative Criteria:

_____ Properly wash hands
_____ Use proper technique using equipment in home
_____ Introduce self to patient
_____ Ask for current status since last visit

_____ Converse in a clinically appropriate way
_____ Perform thorough cardiovascular and wound assessment
_____ Proceed in a logical and organized manner
_____ Determine that wound is infected
_____ Convey finding to peers, patient or caregiver, and primary nurse
_____ Call physician
_____ Recognize that he or she is not able to take a verbal order from the physician
_____ Redress wound
_____ Explain next steps to patient or caregiver
_____ Wash hands

G. Debriefing Guidelines

Instructor may debrief with the students in the small group or may use the scenario as a learning experience for the larger classroom. The focus of the debriefing is on the students' perception of the visit, including comfort and accuracy of assessment; communications with patient, peers, primary nurse, and physicians; and anticipatory planning and discussion with patient or caregiver.

Questions used for debriefing with students:

1. Generally speaking, what is your assessment of your home visit to this patient?
2. If you could do the visit over, what would you do differently?
3. Throughout the process of providing care, where was your focus? (If their focus was on the wound care, how aware were they of the situation of the patient?)
4. Please explain how the assessment of the patient's cardiovascular status relates to the condition of the wound.
5. What other assessments are warranted based on the presence of infection?
6. How confident were you in your verbal and written communications?
7. If you were making the next home visit tomorrow, what would you emphasize and why?

H. Suggestions/Key Features to Replicate or Improve

The key concepts here are communications in verbal and written formats, assessment of cardiovascular and wound status, and performance of a wound redressing in a home care setting. This scenario can be easily adapted for use in an acute-care setting and/or used in a medical-surgical nursing course to emphasize continuity of care from hospital to home.

I. Recommendations for Further Use

One of the advantages of running this scenario in a home setting is that it removes some of the institutional supports that students (and nurses!) tend to rely on. Usually, the resources available to the home care nurse are limited. The dressings are limited to those in the home; the telephone may be the only contact to the instructor, the primary nurse, and/or the primary care provider; and the lack of additional supports requires creativity. Additional challenges can be introduced by having the family speak a foreign language, having no caregiver present, or having the primary care provider be inaccessible.

Reference

National Council of State Boards of Nursing. (2007). *NCLEX-RN examination: Test plan for the National Council Licensure Examination for Registered Nurses*. Retrieved June 18, 2008, from https://www.ncsbn.org/RN_Test_Plan_2007_Web.pdf

Recommended Readings

Ebersole, P., Hess, P., & Luggen, A. (2004). *Toward healthy aging: Human needs and nursing responses* (6th ed.). St. Louis, MO: Mosby/Elsevier.

Lewis, S., Heitkemper, M., Dirksen, S., O'Brien, P., & Bucher, L. (2007). *Medical surgical nursing: Assessment & management of clinical problems* (7th ed). St. Louis, MO: Mosby/Elsevier.

Web Sites

Prevention Plus (http://www.bradenscale.com/bradenscale.htm). Provides tools for skin assessment and rating of pressure ulcers.

Wound Care Information Network (http://medicaledu.com/default.htm). A useful site for clinical information related to all aspects of wound care.

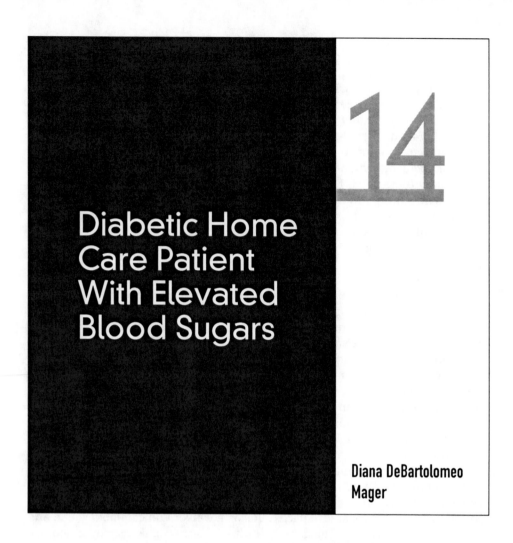

14

Diabetic Home Care Patient With Elevated Blood Sugars

Diana DeBartolomeo
Mager

A & B. Discussion of Implementation of Simulation-Based Pedagogy in Each Contributor's Individualized Teaching and Description of Educational Materials Available in Your Teaching Area and Relative to Your Specialty

In my role as the director of the Robin Kanarek Learning Resource Center at Fairfield University, I have taught a range of nursing skills using a variety of methods. There is a world of difference between using a step-by-step approach to teaching (e.g., when teaching a basic nursing skill like giving an injection) and using a simulated scenario to integrate learning (e.g., having a patient tell the student to get out of the room when he or she approaches the patient to give the injection). I have found it more challenging and time-consuming to set up and run simulations efficiently than to simply teach skills using a step-by-step approach.

Using simulations as a teaching method requires a great deal of forethought. Clear learning objectives and debriefing guidelines need to be set ahead of time. Students must be aware of the objectives and be comfortable with the content that will be addressed during the scenario. Equipment needs to be gathered, set up, and used in a practice run before the live scenario takes place. The practice run requires that faculty members, any volunteers who will role play in the scenario, and student volunteers be present at the same time in order to make sure that there are no "bugs" in the system! Housekeeping issues such as "Is the room available when I want to use it?" need to be thought out ahead as well. Finally, there needs to be some mechanism of evaluation after the scenario is run. When the planning, set up, and practice go well, the running of the simulation may look effortless to others who are watching. At times, this has created an illusion that one can quickly decide to do a simulation and like magic it appears and runs smoothly! In reality, it is not magic but merely sound planning and preparation.

I have assisted faculty members in both writing and running different scenarios for various courses. Many of the initial simulations were created using a high-fidelity human patient simulator (HPS) but without setting up or programming the scenario into the computer. One person controls the HPS based on the activities that the students initiate as they happen. This method has been called running the scenario "on the fly," and it works effectively once the handler knows the controls and software comfortably. In addition, most of the initial scenarios created were designed to simulate the acute-care setting. Because my background is in community health, the following scenario is an attempt at creating a home care situation, and it incorporates the possibility of role-play with or without the need for a HPS.

Although created as a home care scenario, this simulation experience can be easily modified to fit into an acute- or long-term care setting as well. The Resource Center has a small area designed to accommodate home care scenarios. It simulates a small bedroom of an older adult and houses a twin bed, bedside table, television set, assistive devices such as a walker and commode chair, and small props such as vases, magazines, tissue boxes, eyeglasses, and a denture cup. For this scenario, it is feasible to place an HPS into the bed and answer the student's questions through a microphone or to utilize a volunteer to act as the patient. Because our home care room is limited in size, only a small group of students are able to view or participate in a home care scenario at one time. A video recording device is used to record the scenario so that it can be used to debrief or to teach a larger classroom audience at a later date.

C. Specific Objective for Simulation Utilization Within a Specific Course and the Overall Program

The overall objective of this scenario is that the student performs a history and physical examination in a home care setting. In addition, the student demonstrates critical thinking skills in order to link an acute illness with hyperglycemia (Lewis, Heitkemper, Dirksen, O'Brien, & Butcher, 2007, p. 1272). In this scenario, the abnormal findings are urinary frequency and burning, and the daughter has left a note with a list of elevated blood sugars. This simulation may be utilized within the context of a number of different courses, including health assessment, community health, and medical-surgical nursing.

D. Introduction of Scenario to Include Setting the Scene, Technology Used, Objectives, and Description of Participants

Setting the Scene and Technology Used

The scene takes place in the home of an older adult. The patient's daughter has called the home care agency and reported that her mother's blood sugars have been elevated for the past few days, but other than that, her mother feels fine. The patient is due for a nursing visit that day, and the student nurse is going to make the visit.

The patient can be either a volunteer (another student, a faculty member, lab director) or an HPS, dressed in a nightgown and lying in a bed with a walker nearby. Personal items are near the bed, such as glasses, a tissue box, magazines, and the patient's glucometer. A daughter who lives with the patient has left a list of recent elevated blood sugar results on the table near the patient for the nurse to see. There is a phone so that the student may call the physician with pertinent findings. One may or may not give the student a written health history form to simulate forms that would be present in a home care situation.

If using an HPS in the scenario, the person running the scenario may answer questions for the patient as appropriate. However, if a volunteer is utilized, the scenario can be run with very little technology and be quite successful.

Objectives

The overall objectives for this scenario are that the student will: obtain a health history in a home care setting and will use critical thinking skills to differentiate abnormal from normal findings. In addition, the student will decide on the appropriate course of action to take, relating the abnormal findings to the patients uncontrolled diabetes.

The National Council Licensure Examination for a Registered Nurse (NCLEX-RN) test plan categories and subcategories (NCSBN, 2007) addressed in the simulation are as follows:

Safe and Effective Care Environment
Management of Care
Case Management
Collaboration With Interdisciplinary Team
Establishing Priorities
Safety and Infection Control
Handling Hazardous and Infectious Materials
Medical and Surgical Asepsis
Standard/Transmission-based/Other Precautions
Health Promotion and Maintenance
Principles of Teaching/Learning
Techniques of Physical Assessment
Psychosocial Integrity
Family Dynamics
Support Systems

Physiological Integrity
> Basic Care and Comfort
>> Elimination
>> Nutrition and Oral Hydration
> Reduction of Risk Potential
>> Laboratory Values
>> Potential for Alterations in Body Systems
>> Therapeutic Procedures (Finger Stick)
> Physiological Adaptation
>> Illness Management
>> Infectious Diseases
>> Pathophysiology

Description of Participants

1. *Student nurse in community health rotation:* The student should be prepared in the proper use of bag technique for a home care setting. He or she should have had a health assessment course and content relating to both urinary tract infection as well as diabetes. A health history recording form may be given to the student as a guide, but the student should be prepared to ask pertinent questions to the patient. It is up to the student to ask questions in a logical order and use terminology that the patient can understand.
2. *Older adult in the home care setting:* The older adult should be lying down, dressed in a nightgown with a shawl around the shoulders, and with personal items surrounding her. She should tend to answer questions in a lengthy manner and stray off of topic so that the student has to redirect her in order to get the necessary information. The patient should not volunteer a lot of information about urinary symptoms unless specifically asked by the student.
3. *Instructor running the scenario:* The person running the scenario has very little to do other than speak for the simulator if using high-fidelity technology. If a volunteer is being used instead, the instructor is there to observe and record if and how the objectives are being met. In addition, notes may be kept that will aid in debriefing later.

E. Describe Running of the Scenario

Prior to the scenario, the student is given information describing the setting as well as a report about the patient's past and current history. The student may or may not be given a recording sheet to guide him or her in performing the history and physical examination. A home care nursing bag should be provided to the student. Materials in the bag include handwashing supplies, a thermometer, a blood pressure cuff and stethoscope, alcohol wipes, gloves, and a urine culture cup with biohazard lab bags. The patient will have her own glucometer with necessary supplies, a list of recent blood sugars, and a note from the daughter at the bedside. After making an introduction, the student should begin the visit by doing the history and physical exam.

F. Presentation of Completed Template

Title: Diabetic Home Care Patient With Elevated Blood Sugars

Focus Area: Nursing 330, Community Health, Health Assessment, and Medical-Surgical Nursing

Scenario Desciption: This scenario will take place in the home of an older adult female patient who has a history of well-controlled diabetes and is presenting with recent elevated blood sugars. Students will be expected to perform a head-to-toe physical assessment as well as record a thorough health history.

Scenario Objectives:

1. The student will perform a head-to-toe physical assessment on an older adult in a home care setting.
2. The student will obtain and record a health history from an older adult in a home care setting.
3. The student will utilize critical thinking skills on discovering an abnormal finding in the health history (urinary frequency and burning) by deciding on a course of action.
4. The student will utilize critical thinking skills to relate an abnormal finding to an elevation in blood sugars.

Setting the Scene:

> *Equipment needed:* HPS or volunteer; video recording device (optional); home care nursing bag carrying handwashing supplies, thermometer, blood pressure cuff and stethoscope, alcohol wipes, gloves, and a urine culture cup with biohazard lab bags; glucometer; note from daughter with recent blood sugars on it; bed; props to simulate a home care area; health history recording form; telephone
>
> *Resources needed:* Health assessment textbook or community health textbook
>
> *Simulator level:* Human volunteer or HPS
>
> *Participants needed:* A student nurse making the visit, a volunteer as home care patient if not using HPS, and a person running and/or observing the scenario

Scenario Implementation: A simulated home care area can be created in a classroom by rolling in an armed chair and covering it with a quilt and placing any small table next to it.

Required Student Assessments and Actions

Proper handwashing; ability to introduce self to patient; ability to ask pertinent questions when taking a health history; ability to perform head-to-toe physical examination; awareness of the need to check the note at the bedside; ability to report urinary symptoms and obtain an order for a urine culture

Instructor Interventions

Answering the health history questions for the patient if using a high-fidelity HPS; acting as the physician on the phone if the student decides to call the physician

Evaluative Criteria:

_____ Properly wash hands
_____ Use proper bag technique
_____ Introduce self to patient
_____ Look at recent blood sugar note from daughter
_____ Obtain thorough health history
_____ Ask pertinent questions in general
_____ Ask questions so patient can understand
_____ Perform thorough physical examination
_____ History and physical are logically organized
_____ Acknowledge urinary symptoms
_____ State that he or she will check a random blood sugar
_____ Able to state normal and abnormal blood sugar values when patient asks
_____ Ask about diet
_____ Call physician
_____ State that he or she will obtain a urine specimen
_____ Explain symptoms to the patients
_____ Link possibility that urinary symptoms are related to elevated blood sugars
_____ Wash hands
_____ Make attempt to contact daughter in some manner (note, call, etc.) (BONUS)

G. Debriefing Guidelines

Instructor may debrief with the student individually or may use the scenario as a learning experience for the larger classroom.

Questions used for debriefing:

1. How did you plan/prepare for your homecare visit? What kinds of things did you look up, and what references did you use?
2. What did you think when you walked in and saw the patient in the bed?
3. How important was the daughter's note to you?
4. What were you thinking as your patient was giving long answers that were not always on target?
5. What are some ways that you can redirect a patient who is not answering your questions?
6. What did you think when the patient reported urinary frequency and burning?
7. What are normal blood sugar values?
8. What are some other things that can make a diabetic's blood sugars elevate?
9. What else could you have explained or taught to the patient?

H. Suggestions/Key Features to Replicate or Improve

The key concepts here are history taking and performance of a physical examination in a home care setting. However, the scenario can be easily adapted for use in an acute-care setting and used in medical-surgical nursing courses.

I. Recommendations for Further Use

Often, home care nursing visits are complicated and time-consuming due to any number of factors. Depending on the length of time available to run the scenario, as well as the level of the students participating, one could add great detail to replicate real-life dilemmas. For example, socioeconomic issues could be introduced by having the patient state that she is unable to afford antibiotics for her infection; psycho-social issues could arise as the patient states that she is afraid to complain about her health for fear that she will be placed in a long-term care facility; or spiritual issues may occur as a patient states that there is nothing left to live for.

J. Discussion of Simulation-Based Pedagogy and How This New Technology Has Contributed to Improved Student Outcomes

As the director of the Resource Center, I have seen both faculty and students embrace simulation with cautious enthusiasm! Once the initial intimidation of using a new teaching method passes, the usefulness of simulation shines through and is appreciated. Students have been very willing to volunteer to participate in a simulation while their actions are projected onto a larger screen in a nearby room for all their classmates to see in real time. Faculty members have been wonderful about using tactful yet pertinent feedback to make the simulation comfortable for participants and valuable for the student audience. The use of simulation-based pedagogy allows students to perform nursing care in a risk-free environment while adding interest and excitement to the classroom.

References

Lewis, S., Heitkemper, M., Dirksen, S., O'Brien, P., & Bucher, L. (2007). *Medical surgical nursing: Assessment & management of clinical problems* (7th ed). St. Louis, MO: Mosby Elsevier.

National Council of State Boards of Nursing. (2007). *NCLEX-RN examination: Test plan for the National Council Licensure Examination for Registered Nurses.* Retrieved April 14, 2007, from https://www.ncsbn.org/RN_Test_Plan_2007_Web.pdf

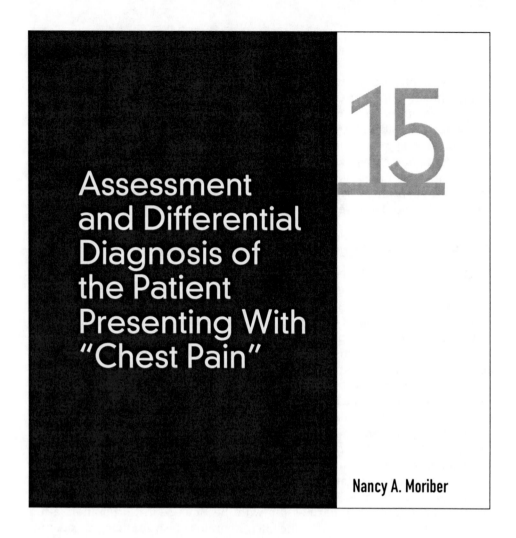

15

Assessment and Differential Diagnosis of the Patient Presenting With "Chest Pain"

Nancy A. Moriber

A. Discussion of Implementation of Simulation-Based Pedagogy in Each Contributor's Individualized Teaching

The use of simulation in nurse anesthesia training has been an integral part of the educational process for many years. As an educator, I have been using low-fidelity simulation and static trainers to teach basic psychomotor skills and critical decision making since taking on the role of program director for the Fairfield University and Bridgeport Hospital Nurse Anesthesia Program 4 years ago. However, with the addition of high-fidelity simulation, the nurse anesthesia program has been able to move to the next level and incorporate the simulation-based pedagogy of the Fairfield University School of Nursing throughout the curriculum. Scenarios are utilized in the student's clinical orientation and in all five clinical practica in order to facilitate the progression from novice to competent anesthesia care provider. High-fidelity simulation introduces students to situations that are rarely encountered in the clinical setting but in which expertise is essential for safe practice. Since my area of expertise is in graduate education, the following scenario will be applicable to senior-level undergraduate and entry-level advanced practice students.

This chapter will focus on the assessment, differential diagnosis, and initial treatment of the patient who presents to the Emergency Department (ED) with complaints of crushing substernal chest pain. The student will be required to conduct a rapid history and physical, develop an initial diagnosis, initiate lifesaving therapy, and utilize effective communication techniques with the patient, family, and members of the interdisciplinary health care team in order to successfully meet the objectives of the scenario. The scenario can be modified for use in the primary care, intensive care, medical-surgical, or perioperative setting as required to meet the specific needs of the students.

B. Description of Educational Materials Available in Your Teaching Area and Relative to Your Specialty

The Fairfield University School of Nursing Robin Kanarek Learning Resource Center (LRC) is a state-of-the-art facility designed to foster the development of psychomotor, cognitive, and affective clinical skills in our students. It is equipped with two simulation rooms that have been set up to simulate an intensive care or operative environment. The simulation rooms share a control room that is capable of recording and transmitting in real-time running scenarios to adjacent classrooms in order to facilitate effective debriefing.

Either simulation room can be utilized to run the proposed scenario because the necessary equipment is readily available to the instructor in each area including, but not limited to, cardiac and respiratory monitors, a head wall with oxygen and suction, medication carts, cardiac defibrillators, an EKG machine, and appropriate resuscitative equipment. The equipment necessary to conduct a physical assessment is also available within the LRC. In addition, as a result of the School of Nursing partnership with the Emergisoft Corporation, a full database of patient records that includes laboratory tests, radiologic examinations, and EKGs will be available to enhance the educational opportunities of the scenario.

C. Specific Objective for Simulation Utilization Within a Specific Course and the Overall Program

The overarching objectives of this scenario are threefold and are consistent with both the program essentials for undergraduate and graduate education as delineated by the American Association of Colleges of Nursing (AACN, 1996, 1998). This scenario will enhance the student's ability to do the following:

1. Collaborate with peers, patients, health care professionals, and other members of the health care team in the assessment, planning, implementation, and evaluation of health care.
2. Utilize critical thinking skills and current scientific evidence in the clinical decision-making process.
3. Communicate effectively in order to provide appropriate patient-centered care.

This scenario is designed for undergraduate nursing students who have completed their basic medical-surgical experience and are participating in transitional experiences in critical care settings during their senior year. It can also be utilized at the graduate level as part of the advanced-practice nursing curriculum in the Advanced Health Assessment or Advanced Physiology and Pathophysiology courses.

D. Introduction of Scenario to Include Setting the Scene, Technology Used, Objectives, and Description of Participants

Setting the Scene:
This scenario takes place in the ED. The patient has just walked into the waiting room with her husband and tells the nurse at the triage desk that she has had crushing substernal chest pain that has been radiating to her back for the past hour and has not been relieved by rest. She was out for dinner with her husband at their favorite local Italian restaurant prior to the onset of symptoms. She states that she feels "terrible." Her husband is very anxious and insistent that something be done for his wife immediately. The patient is placed in a room with a monitored bed, where the ED nurse (student) that will be caring for her is waiting. This is where the scenario begins.

Technology Used
In order to run this scenario, a high-fidelity human patient simulator (HPS) simulator will be utilized so that the student can visualize hemodynamic and EKG changes that will be implemented as part of the scenario. If one is not available, an actor can be substituted, but the instructors will need to get more creative with displaying hemodynamic changes. Access to patient records, either in electronic or paper format, will also be necessary. Electronic records will allow for greater scenario realism, as the majority of EDs have gone to electronic formatting for patient medical records. Audio-taped recordings of the common sounds in the ED will also be incorporated into the scenario to simulate the noisy and hectic emergency environment. Finally, video recording equipment will be required to tape the scenario so that it can be evaluated and discussed during debriefing sessions. It is important to note that when implementing video recording of student performance, written permission is required and should be obtained at the start of the simulation session or, ideally, on entrance into the program. A blanket release form can be used to cover all simulation sessions in which a student participates during his or her educational experience.

Specific Scenario Objectives and National Council Licensure Examination for a Registered Nurse Target Areas
At the completion of this scenario, the student will be able to do the following:

1. Discuss the differential diagnosis of "life-threatening" chest pain.
2. Conduct an immediate targeted physical assessment and health history.

3. Initiate intravenous fluid therapy.
4. Discuss possible alternative diagnoses in the patient presenting with chest pain, including noncardiac (gastroesophageal reflux disease) and vascular causes.
5. Discuss the initial treatment of acute coronary syndrome (ACS), including the drugs, dosages, and adjuvant treatment modalities.
6. Apply the advanced cardiac life support (ACLS) ACS algorithm.
7. Interpret common laboratory and diagnostic tests utilized in the differential diagnosis of ACS, including cardiac enzymes, troponin levels, and the EKG.
8. Develop skills as a team leader, patient advocate, and effective communicator.

National Council Licensure Examination for a Registered Nurse (NCLEX-RN) test plan categories and subcategories (NCSBN, 2007) addressed in this scenario include the following:

Safe and Effective Care Environment
    Management of Care
        Case Management
        Collaboration with Interdisciplinary Team
        Consultation
        Establishing Priorities
        Resource Management
    Safety and Infection Control
        Handling Hazardous and Infectious Materials
        Safe Use of Equipment
        Standard/Transmission-Based/Other Precautions
Health Promotion and Maintenance
        Techniques of Physical Assessment
Psychosocial Integrity
        Crisis Intervention
        Family Dynamics
        Situational Role Changes
        Support Systems
        Therapeutic Communications
Physiological Integrity
    Pharmacological and Parenteral Therapies
        Dosage Calculation
        Expected Effects/Outcomes
        Medication Administration
        Parenteral/Intravenous Therapies
        Pharmacological Agents/Actions
    Reduction of Risk Potential
        Diagnostic Tests
        Laboratory Values
        Potential for Alterations in Body System

Therapeutic Procedures
Vital Signs
Physiological Adaptation
Alterations in Body Systems
Hemodynamics
Medical Emergencies
Pathophysiology

Description of Participants

A total of five participants will be required to run this scenario properly. The student to be evaluated will take the role of the ED nurse assessing the patient. He or she will be given the role of team leader and will be required to delegate tasks and coordinate interdisciplinary discussion and activities. The student should have completed the didactic module on the care of the patient with ACS and should have a solid foundation in pharmacology, including pharmacokinetics, pharmacodynamics, and drug side effects. The student must also have completed a basic health assessment course, received prior training in the institution of intravenous therapy, and must have completed content on the interpretation of basic laboratory and diagnostic tests. An assessment form may be given to the student to help guide the scenario, if deemed appropriate by the instructors.

A second student or actor can take on the role of the nursing technician (or the equivalent). This individual is included to serve as member of the health care team and will be required to carry out tasks as directed by the ED nurse. This can include such tasks as sending blood to the lab, obtaining equipment, or assisting with procedures. The purpose is to assess the student's ability to delegate and work as a member of the health care team.

An actor (or student) will be needed to serve as the patient's husband. This individual should be provided with a short script and a description of the scene so that he can effectively portray the anxious husband. This individual should not offer any information about the patient unless specifically asked. The husband is included to facilitate communication and activation of support systems.

Role of the Husband

1. *The scene:* Mr. Hart brings his wife, Mrs. Hart, to the ED with complaints of crushing substernal chest pain that radiates to her back and has lasted more than an hour. The couple was out for dinner at their favorite local Italian restaurant prior to the onset of the symptom, and they consumed a very heavy meal. Mr. Hart is extremely anxious and is demanding that his wife be seen immediately. He is yelling at the nurses and ancillary staff and is being disruptive to other patients in the waiting room.
2. *Suggested dialogue:*
   a. If Mr. Hart's needs are not addressed:
      i. "My wife needs help, and I want it now!"
      ii. "Somebody do something now, or I'll take her inside myself!"

      iii. Don't tell me to calm down! You don't have any idea how I feel right now."

      iv. If you don't do something now, you are going to have two patients to take care of!"

  b. If appropriate intervention occurs (involvement of family support services, reassurance provided):

      i. "Oh, thank you so much. I knew somebody would care."

      ii. You are all so wonderful, I know my wife is in good hands!"

      iii. Will you keep me informed of what is going on? We've been together for 40 years, and I don't know what I would do without her."

Finally, two faculty members will be required. One faculty member will run the simulation and act as the voice of the patient, and the other will serve as the ED physician and will be imbedded in the scenario. If a second faculty member is not available, a student/actor can be utilized, but it is necessary to realize that no one will be available to help facilitate movement and guide the student through the scenario should it become necessary. The purpose of the ED physician is to act as a collaborating member of the health care team. The scenario can be modified if desired and the ED physician portrayed in a confrontational fashion, thereby allowing assessment of the student's abilities to handle stressful situations, resolve conflict, and improve communication. If there are no faculty members or students available to play the role of the physician, the individual running the scenario could as a last resort portray the physician utilizing a telephone consult format. This could help refine the student's communication skills, with particular attention paid to confirming the accuracy of understanding between scenario participants.

E. Describe Running of the Scenario

Prior to running the scenario, the student must complete the didactic component required to effectively manage the scenario. This includes a complete discussion of the management of ACS as outlined in the ACLS professional provider's manual (American Heart Association, 2006). In addition, the student should also have completed his or her course work in advanced physiology and pathophysiology. The students should be made aware of the general purpose of the scenario—the differential diagnosis of chest pain—prior to attending the simulation session. In addition, the students will be provided with an ED health history and nursing record in order to familiarize themselves with the requirements. If an electronic database is available, the students must be trained in the proper use of the system so that troubleshooting the electronic record does not become the focus of the scenario. All necessary equipment will be in the simulation room, including a stethoscope, EKG machine, defibrillator, medication cart, all necessary "mock" oral and intravenous medications, oxygen therapy, and all materials necessary for the insertion of an intravenous line. Finally, all participants except the ED nurse should be readily available but not at the patient's bedside so that the student's ability to utilize resources can be assessed. The scenario will begin when the triage nurse (the instructor) informs the ED nurse that Mrs. Hart is being admitted to bed #5.

F. Presentation of Completed Template

Title: Assessment and Differential Diagnosis of the Patient Presenting With "Chest Pain"

Focus Area:
Advanced health assessment

Scenario Description:
Mrs. Hart is a 54-year-old female who presents to the ED complaining of crushing substernal chest pain that radiates to her back. It began approximately 1 hour prior to admission and has not been relieved with rest. She was out for dinner with her husband at their favorite local Italian restaurant prior to the onset of symptoms. Her husband, who is extremely anxious and is demanding that his wife be seen immediately, accompanies her.

Her past medical history is significant for hypertension × 3 years that has been well controlled as well as noninsulin-dependent diabetes mellitus. Her medications include metoprolol (Lopressor) 50 mg po twice a day, lisinopril (Prinivil, Zestril) 10 mg po once a day, and metformin (Glucophage) 500 mg po twice a day. She has no known drug allergies. Surgical history is positive for a tonsillectomy and adenoidectomy as a child.

Scenario Objectives:

1. Discuss the differential diagnosis of "life-threatening" versus chest discomfort.
2. Conduct an immediate targeted physical assessment and health history.
3. Initiate intravenous therapy.
4. Discuss possible alternative diagnoses in the patient presenting with chest pain, including noncardiac (gastroesophageal reflux disease) and vascular causes.
5. Discuss the initial treatment of ACS, including the drugs, dosages, and adjuvant treatment modalities.
6. Apply the ACLS ACS algorithm.
7. Develop skills as a team leader, patient advocate, and effective communicator.

Setting the Scene:

Equipment needed:
High-fidelity simulator; video recording device; patient monitor; blood pressure cuff; EKG; pulse oximeter; oxygen flow meter; nasal cannula and face mask; intravenous line; intravenous insertion kit; intravenous pole; blood drawing equipment; medications including morphine, aspirin, nitroglycerine, and heparin; and ED patient record (medical)

Resources needed:
Laboratory reports including CBC and troponin levels and computer access if laboratory reports are to be posted within a database; ACLS provider manual

Simulator level:
High-fidelity simulation

Participants needed:

Five participants required: emergency room nurse (student role), nursing technician (student/actor), ED physician (faculty member imbedded in the scenario), faculty member to operate high-fidelity simulator, actor to play patient's anxious husband

A small part should be scripted for the role of the husband if the actor is a nonfaculty member.

Scenario Implementation:

Initial Settings for High-Fidelity Simulator

BP: 168/90, HR: 110 beats per minute, RR: 28, oxygen saturation: 98%

Required Student Assessments and Actions

1. Reassure husband, identify staff member/hospital representative to attend to his needs.
2. Within the first 10 minutes, the student should implement immediate assessment and general treatment as follows:
   a. Check vital signs, including blood pressure, heart rate, respiratory rate; evaluates oxygen saturation.
   b. Start oxygen at 4 L per minute to keep oxygen saturation above 90%.
   c. Establish IV access.
   d. Give aspirin (Bayer, Excedrin) 160–325 mg, nitroglycerine (Tridil) sublingual or spray, and morphine IV as appropriate.
      i. Identify need to use nitroglycerine (Tridil)/morphine cautiously in the patient who is hypotensive or bradycardic.
      ii. Perform brief, targeted history and physical examination.
      iii. Note onset of symptoms, associated or precipitating factors, and timing and sequence of symptoms.
   e. Obtain a 12-lead EKG.
   f. Obtain initial laboratory tests, including troponin, CPK-MB, and electrolyte and coagulation profile.
   g. Identify contraindications for fibrinolytic therapy:
      i. Onset chest discomfort >12 hours, pre-existing coagulapathy, recent cerebral vascular event or trauma, severe systemic hypertension, pregnancy, history of structural CNS disease or severe systemic disease.
   h. Order chest x-ray.
3. Review EKG and cardiac enzymes with physician.
   a. If EKG normal or nondiagnostic and troponin levels normal, identifies patient as low risk for unstable angina.
      i. Order serial cardiac markers, observation, repeat EKG.
      ii. Consider other possible causes of chest pain, including GI and vascular, and reevaluates patient's history.
         (1) Consider GERD/esophageal spasm.
            (a) Spasms may respond to nitroglycerine and lead to inappropriate diagnosis.
         (2) Trial of antacids.
      iii. Discharge patient with appropriate follow-up.

   b. If EKG is abnormal, demonstrating ST segment elevation or depression, refers for appropriate in-house treatment.

      i. ST elevation MI (STEMI) identifies appropriate treatment including beta-adrenergic blockade, heparin, clopidogrel (Plavix) 300 mg po × 1 dose, and reperfusion therapy if not contraindicated.

      ii. High-risk unstable angina or non–ST elevation MI (ST depression) identifies appropriate treatment including nitroglycerine, beta-adrenergic blockade, heparin, clopidogrel (Plavix), and glycoprotein IIb/IIIa inhibitor.

4. Notify husband of patient's condition. Discuss appropriate treatment and follow-up.

Instructor Interventions

The instructor running the simulator will act as the voice of the patient and will answer all questions posed by the student in the scenario. In addition, this faculty member will be required to "run" the simulator and make the appropriate responses, both verbal and hemodynamic, in response to student behaviors. The instructor imbedded within the scenario is there to facilitate student performance and provide guidance in accordance with the terminal objectives of the scenario.

Evaluative Criteria:

Students will be evaluated based on the degree to which they perform in appropriate order, with or without coaching, the actions outlined above (Table 15.1).

G. Debriefing Guidelines

Debriefing is an essential part of the simulation experience, and in many instances, it is the most important learning tool utilized in this teaching/learning pedagogy. In order to get the most out of this experience, it would be beneficial for the scenario to be recorded and then critically examined individually by the students as well as by the class as a whole. Students should be provided with the evaluation criteria outlined above prior to viewing the taped simulation. Questions that can be utilized by the instructor to facilitate discussion should include the following:

1. Overall, how do you think the scenario went? What do you think could have been done differently? What would you do the same?
2. What is the underlying pathophysiology of ACS?
3. What are the differences between an ST elevation MI (STEMI) and a non–ST elevation MI?
4. What are the indications and contraindications for the use of fibrinolytic therapy in the setting of an acute MI?
5. What are the most commonly used drugs for the treatment of ACS and what are the most common side effects?
6. What are the normal and abnormal values for cardiac enzyme lab values?
7. What are some of the barriers to effective treatment of the patient presenting with ACS?

15.1 Evaluating Student Criteria in a Nursing Simulation Scenario			
Behavior	Independent	Prompting	Appropriate Order
Reassure husband			
Assess vital signs			
Apply oxygen 4 L/minute			
Establish IV access			
Administer aspirin, nitroglycerine, morphine in appropriate doses			
Perform brief, targeted history			
Initial assessment carried out in <10 minutes			
Obtain 12-lead EKG			
Obtain appropriate laboratory tests			
Identify contraindications to fibrinolytic therapy			
Order chest X-ray			
Review labs, EKG, and follows ACS protocol a. EKG normal, nondiagnostic: Considers other possibilities, including GERD, esophageal spasm, repeat EKG, serial enzyme b. EKG abnormal, follows ST elevation (STEMI), non–ST elevation (ST depression) protocol			
Notify husband of patient's status			
Work as a member of the health care team			

IV, intravenous; EKG, electrocardiogram; ACS, acute coronary syndrome; GERD, gastroesophageal reflux disease.

8. How can you (as the ED nurse) facilitate communication and collaboration among members of the interdisciplinary health care team?
9. How did the presence of the patient's husband alter the care provided to the patient in this situation?
10. Do you think the husband's needs are a priority in this situation? Why or why not? Whose responsibility is it to see that they are met?
11. What are some of the other possible causes of "chest pain" in this patient? How do you make the differential diagnosis?

H & I. Suggestions/Key Features to Replicate or Improve and Recommendations for Further Use

Understanding the physiologic principles and key aspects of the ACLS ACS algorithm is essential prior to the execution of this scenario. As patient scenarios become more advanced and incorporate a multitude of physiologic and pharmacologic principles, utilizing a variety of experiential learning techniques to reinforce key principles could enhance learning. Providing in-class didactic instruction that incorporates computer-based simulation programs such as Laerdal's MicroSim® would be extremely useful because it provides the student with beginning opportunities to practice critical decision making and make clinical judgments in a less-threatening learning environment. Instructor feedback and class debriefing can enhance learning in this situation as well.

This scenario can also be modified and the differential diagnosis changed to further enhance the student's health assessment skills. For example, in the scenario outlined above, the patient presenting with chest pain could have had a dissecting thoracic aneurysm, severe esophagitis, or pleuritic chest pain. While each condition would present with similar symptoms, there are key differences that could be explored in the scenario, therefore sending the student down a different path. By allowing students to explore different diagnoses, they will be able to improve both their physical assessment skills and their ability to utilize clinical evidence in the decision-making process.

J. Discussion of Simulation-Based Pedagogy and How This New Technology Has Contributed to Improved Student Outcomes

Students enjoy utilizing simulation as a learning tool. It provides them with the opportunity to develop psychomotor, cognitive, and affective skills in a less-threatening and safe environment. It also enables educators to expose students to a greater repertoire of clinical situations than would normally be encountered during the course of education and training. Adopting a simulation-based pedagogy and incorporating simulation throughout the curriculum enables educators to expose students to a variety of complicated and challenging situations that can only improve the quality of care provided by graduates. In addition, as methods of evaluating student performance improve, simulation can be used to guide clinical remediation and even clinical advancement. The opportunities are endless. It only takes motivation, creativity, and a commitment to improving the quality of education provided to our students.

References

American Association of Colleges of Nursing. (1998). *Essentials of master's education for advanced practice nursing*. Washington, DC: AACN.

American Association of Colleges of Nursing. (1998). *Essentials of baccalaureate education for professional nursing practice*. Washington, DC: AACN.

American Heart Association. (2006). *Advanced cardiovascular life support: Professional provider manual*. Dallas: American Heart Association.

National Council of State Boards of Nursing. (2007). *NCLEX-RN examination: Test plan for the national council licensure examination for registered nurses*. Retrieved September 2, 2008, from https://www.ncsbn.org/RN_Test_Plan_2007_Web.pdf

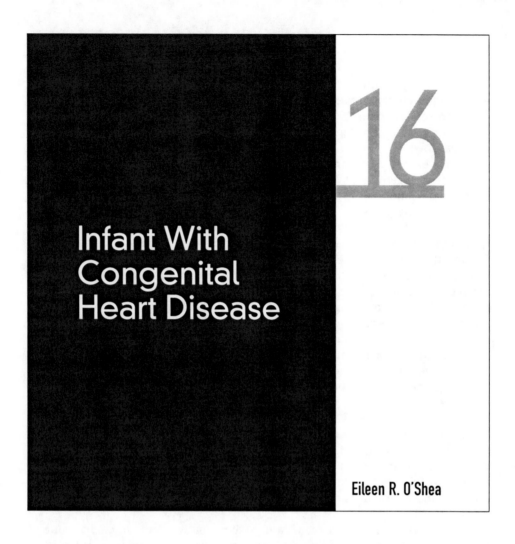

16

Infant With Congenital Heart Disease

Eileen R. O'Shea

This chapter will explore the care of the infant with congenital heart disease who has received palliative cardiac surgery. Priority physiologic goals for this simulation include decreasing cardiac output, promoting effective breathing, and managing nutritional needs. The principle of providing "bundle or cluster care" for the cardiac infant will be incorporated into the scenario along with the philosophy of family-centered care. An emphasis is placed on organizing care so that the student will decrease cardiac output demands by allowing the infant uninterrupted periods of rest (Ball & Bindler, 2008; Hockenberry & Wilson, 2007). Students will need to conduct physical assessments, perform nutritional interventions, and coordinate care with members of the interdisciplinary health care team. Additionally, students will interact with either a single teen parent or the grandmother of the infant.

A. Discussion of Implementation of Simulation-Based Pedagogy in Each Contributor's Individualized Teaching

Adding an interactive component or simulation to a pediatric undergraduate course does not have to be a daunting event. It does not require the purchase of high-fidelity manikins. The purpose of simulated learning is to provide an educational activity for the student without the constraints of a real-life situation (Oermann & Gaberson, 2006). Simulated learning can occur with role-play, skits, or other interactive strategies where students actually take an active part in their own learning.

In my experience, transitioning students from presenting PowerPoint case studies to interactive skits and role-play has led to increased satisfaction among many, as documented by course evaluations. To get to this point, however, was quite a learning process.

As a first-year faculty member, I had utilized many PowerPoint presentations and outlines while teaching pediatric nursing to undergraduate students. I found that students often were not well prepared for class, partly because I did not have a mechanism to hold them accountable for their own learning. During future semesters, I altered my teaching methods to incorporate case studies. My goal was to increase student accountability for their own learning and enhance interaction among the class. What I found was that requiring students to present a case study to their classmates did not guarantee class interaction. In fact, I learned that students resented the "dry, PowerPoint presentations" delivered by their peers. Students described the case study presentations as boring and not contributing to learning, as noted in critiques at the end of the semester.

The next semester, I tried a different approach to student presentations. Rather than abandon the case study method, I altered how the presentations would be evaluated. I required the students to make the cases interactive. The students were to be creative and foster class participation in order to receive full credit. Skits and games were allowed, and nursing research and evidenced practices were required to be integrated into their presentations.

At first, students were reluctant to be creative and to be in front of the class, but once they got started, classes were transformational. Students were responsible, well prepared, and respectful of one another's presentations. Many course evaluations stated that case studies were fun and that students learned a lot while creating and researching their topics. Additionally, I found that the cases and skits fostered group process and collaboration among peers.

B. Description of Educational Materials Available in Your Teaching Area and Relative to Your Specialty

Pediatric educational materials available for our course include both the child and baby static manikins. In addition, I have developed a "pediatric" box of supplies for demonstration purposes. These supplies include items such as neonate, infant, and child blood pressure cuffs; urine bags; feeding tubes; Salem sump tubes; electrocardiogram electrodes; and various other hands on equipment. With a few simple props and targeted case studies, students have created interactive group presentations.

C. Specific Objective for Simulation Utilization Within a Specific Course and the Overall Program

Objectives

Course objectives that are applied within this scenario:

1. Synthesizes knowledge from the arts, sciences, and nursing in the provision of holistic care for children and their families experiencing alterations in health/development.
2. Employs critical thinking skills in analyzing and responding to complex clinical situations.
3. Incorporates supportive and computer-based technology in pediatric nursing care.
4. Collaborates with children, their families, and other health care providers in the planning, delivery, and evaluation of holistic care.
5. Provides and promotes evidence-based, culturally sensitive, and ethically sound nursing care.
6. Demonstrates professional accountability and responsibility in performing all aspects of the nursing student role.

Undergraduate program objectives:

1. Demonstrate effectiveness in planning and providing therapeutic nursing care, managing information, and promoting self-care competence of culturally diverse individuals, families, groups, and communities.
2. Employ a variety of technologies and other therapeutic modalities with sensitivity for the provision of care.
3. Make sound clinical judgments based on nursing science and related theory, using critical thinking and ethical decision making.
4. Demonstrate collaboration with peers, patient, health care professionals, and others within health care teams in the process of planning, delegating, implementing, and evaluating care.
5. Communicate with clarity, purpose, and sensitivity using a variety of methods, including technology.
6. Advocate for patients, consumers, and the nursing profession through involvement in the political process as well as health/patient care policies and practices.

D. Introduction of Scenario to Include Setting the Scene, Technology Used, Objectives, and Description of Participants

Setting the Scene and Technology Used

The scene takes place in an acute-care setting on a general pediatric unit. The infant has had palliative cardiac surgery and has been transferred from the pediatric intensive care unit (PICU) to a general pediatric floor. The infant and family have been assigned a student nurse to provide care for the day shift.

The infant can be a static manikin, baby doll, or a medium-fidelity human patient simulator (HPS) and should be lying in a crib that has been accessorized with infant stimulation toys. The doll should be dressed appropriately, such as with a diaper, onesie tee shirt, socks, and pajamas. Also, electrodes should be attached to the chest, and a pulse oximeter probe should be attached to a toe. There should be supplies on the bedside table to assist with feeding and consoling the infant. Such items may consist of a pacifier, diapers and wipes, syringes, bottle of water, pH paper, and a centimeter tape measure. Outside the infant's room, an area should be arranged for the student to prepare and calculate medicines as well as an area to prepare the infant's formula. The teen mom or the grandmother should be present at the bedside and may or may not have spent the night. This inclusion of the parent/grandmother is to incorporate the principle of family-centered care. The philosophy of family-centered care is to recognize the family as a constant in the child's life and that they are important partners in caring for the hospitalized child (Ball & Bindler, 2008; Hockenberry & Wilson, 2007).

Objectives

1. The student will perform a head-to-toe physical assessment on an infant with congenital heart disease status post cardiothoracic surgery in a pediatric acute-care setting.
2. The student will collaborate and coordinate care with members of an interprofessional health care team.
3. The student will communicate the plan of care to a single teenage mother or to the grandmother.
4. The student will perform appropriate feeding technique for an infant with congenital heart disease.
5. The student will demonstrate accurate placement of a nasogastric (NG) feeding tube, according to hospital policy and as supported by evidence-based practice.
6. The student will demonstrate accurate documentation for an infant with congenital heart disease.

Description of the Participants

1. *Student nurse in general pediatric course:* The student will need to synthesize prior knowledge from previous course work to successfully complete this scenario. Courses such as the Fundamentals of Nursing, Pathopharmacology, Child Development, and Obstetrics will serve as a foundation. An understanding of congenital heart disease and the principle of bundle or cluster care will be important preparation for the learner. He or she should be competent with the following three skills: infant assessment, vital signs, and gavage feeding via an NG tube. A copy of the institution's policy regarding the insertion and verification of placement for NG feeding tubes should be provided. In addition, the student should be comfortable with the philosophy

of family-centered care, and he or she should be informed that there will be a parent at the bedside.

2. *Teen mom or grandmother:* The teen mom is a 16 year old who does not have any other children; she does not work, but is trying to complete high school. If she has slept overnight, then she should be dressed in a hospital gown. An alternative focus for this simulation could include addressing psychosocial needs or health needs of the family. Topics to be considered may include breast-feeding; nutrition and diet of a teen mom; normal child development and infant care; stress of caring for a complex infant; grieving the loss of a well healthy baby; or exploring the relationship with the father of the baby, who has a history of violence.

   Another possibility for this simulation might include the grandmother sitting at the bedside rather than the teen mom. A potential focus of the scenario with this presentation would be for the student to sort through who is the primary caretaker and who will be accountable for the infant once she is discharged to home. Who will the nurse need to include when teaching home care needs? Assessing the grandmother's health and family stressors may be a goal with an intervention of contacting the unit's social worker. Another goal for the student may be to assess where this family gathers support to cope with various stressors, including but not limited to finances, health and illness, work, school, and caring for a medically fragile infant. Spirituality and faith may be a theme that arises, and the student may intervene by contacting pastoral care or the family's home church or faith-based organization.

3. *Clinical instructor:* The clinical instructor should be a faculty person who can assist or prompt the student along the way in order to stay on track with the focus of this scenario being the physiologic needs of the infant. For example, if the focus is feeding the infant, the instructor may prompt the student to leave the room in order to go and prepare while one of the therapists is in the room. Some guidance will keep the scenario running smoothly. The faculty member may also keep anecdotal notes regarding what went well and what may have been done differently, which can be utilized for the debriefing afterwards (Oermann & Gaberson, 2006).

4. *Therapists:* There are two therapists included in this scenario, who can be portrayed by one individual. Initially, the simulation has the respiratory therapist (RT) enter the infant's room to conduct a respiratory assessment and to provide a nebulizer treatment. The RT should be dressed with a lab coat and should bring along a stethoscope, nebulizer, and medication. The student can either ask the RT to stay or come back at another time. The student must coordinate and organize the plan of care. Ideally, the student should use critical thinking skills and recognize that the respiratory treatment will improve the infant's ability to breathe easier and will enhance her ability to feed. The student may also take this time to confer with the RT and review respiratory findings and the plan for the day (i.e., frequency of nebulizers and respiratory goals).

   Once the nebulizer has been administered, the RT leaves, and the occupational therapist (OT) enters the room. The OT may or may not wear a lab coat and should state that he or she has come to work on oral feeding with the infant. The student must coordinate and organize care again with this member of the health care team and may decide to have the OT stay or come back at another time. At this point, the clinical instructor may need to guide or remind the student that time is freed up by utilizing either the OT or the parent at the bedside to administer the oral feeding. The student might want to download and review NG tube care policy or complete documentation at the bedside. The OT can also model the appropriate way to feed this cardiac infant and can use this opportunity to teach the parent best practices for oral feedings. The student should recognize the value of collaborating with a member of the interprofessional health care team. For the more advanced student, medication administration could also be integrated into this scenario, which may be prepared with instructor while the OT works with the mom and infant.

E. Describe Running of the Scenario

The simulation described below focuses on the physiologic needs of this cardiac infant and can be easily altered to be more or less complex, depending on course objectives and the level of the student learner.

To prepare for this simulation, the student should be given a report regarding the infant and information regarding the institution's policy of NG tube insertion and verification of placement. Providing this information 1 week in advance will give the student an opportunity to review content. At our regional children's hospital, the policy to confirm NG tube placement is to aspirate a small amount of stomach contents with a syringe, test the pH, and then measure the length of the tube from the nare to the end. This practice has been supported in the literature and will be utilized in the evaluation of the student (Huffman, Jarczyk, O'Brien, Pieper, & Bayne, 2004; Verger & Lebet, 2008; Westhus, 2004). Once the student has entered the room, an introduction should be made to the mom or grandmother, and a head-to-toe assessment should be performed on the infant, followed by vital signs and a diaper change. After assessments have been completed, the RT should enter the infant's room.

F. Presentation of Completed Template

Title: Infant With Congenital Heart Disease
Nursing of Children and Family (Pediatrics)
Second-semester junior year or first-semester senior year BSN

Focus Area:
Pediatrics

Scenario Description:
The patient is a 4-month-old black female admitted to the general pediatric unit from the PICU status post cardiothoracic surgery for implantation of a shunt due to congenital pulmonary atresia with ventricular septal defect.

> *Secondary diagnoses:* Pulmonary edema; chronic bronchospasm; diaphragm paralysis
> *Patient medical history:* This infant was born at 36 weeks to a 16-year-old single parent.

Immunizations: Up to date

Social: Biologic father of child has history of violence. The teen mom has two older siblings and lives at home with the infant's grandmother. The mother of the child is completing high school. The grandmother is 40 years old and has a history of obesity and hypertension. She works full-time at the local hospital in environmental services. The grandfather of the infant is deceased.

Allergies: NKDA

Medications:

Aspirin, chewable tablet, 20 mg per NG tube once daily

Lansopraxole suspension (Prevacid), 15 mg per NG tube once daily

Metoclopramide syrup (Reglan), 0.5 mg per NG tube every 8 hours

Furosemide (Lasix) tablet, 8 mg per NG tube on empty stomach once daily

Albuterol meter dose inhaler (MDI) with spacer, two inhalations every 4 hours

Height: 57 cm

Weight: 5.1 kg

The infant receives the following care:

VS Q 4 hours and PRN

Accurate I & O

Daily weights

Medications as ordered

Treatments:

Feedings: 95 cc Enfamil with iron, 27 calories per ounce every 3 hours. Begin with oral feeds; administer any remaining formula via NG tube. All feeds (both oral and remainder NG) should be completed within 30 minutes.

Respiratory: Continuous O_2 sat monitoring. Maintain sats >75%. Chest percussion, postural drainage, albuterol nebulizer treatment every 4 hours to relieve bronchospasm to be completed by the RT.

Scenario Objectives:

1. Demonstrate a head-to-toe assessment on an infant.
2. Verify accurate placement of a NG feeding tube.
3. Perform appropriate feeding technique for infant with an NG feeding tube.
4. Document accurate findings for an infant with congenital heart disease.
5. Communicate plan of care to a single teenage mother or grandmother.
6. Collaborate and coordinate care with members of an interdisciplinary health care team.

The American Association of Colleges of Nursing *Essentials of Baccalaureate Education* for Professional Nursing Practice (AACN, 2007) addressed were as follows:

Essential II: Basic Organizational and Systems Leadership, Objectives 1, 5

Essential VI: Interprofessional Communication and Collaboration for Improving Patient Health Outcomes, Objectives 2, 4

Essential IX: Baccalaureate General Nursing Practice, Objectives 1, 3, 5, 7, 11

Setting the Scene:

Patient:
- Baby doll diapered and dressed in a onesie tee shirt.
- #5 Fr. NG feeding tube cut short and secured to cheek with Tegaderm.
- Midline sternal incison can be left open to air or covered with a chest dressing. If left open to air, can use black marker to indicate suture line.
- Pulse oximeter probe attached to the doll's toe and connected to a pulse oximeter monitor.

Equipment needed:
- Crib accessorized with infant stimulation toys (mobile, music, rattles, or soft stuffed animals). If crib is not available, a hospital bed or even the top of a desk could be utilized.
- Pulse oximeter monitor with small toe probe
- Electrocardio patches with electrodes
- Chest percussion device
- Nebulizer
- Albuterol
- Infant face mask
- Stethoscope
- Infant blood pressure cuff
- Thermometer
- Oxygen with flow meter and nasal cannula at head of bed
- NG feeding tube (#5 Fr.)
- pH paper to verify NG placement
- Centimeter paper tape to measure feeding NG tube from tip of nare to end of tube
- 30 or 60 cc syringe for gavage feeding
- 3 cc or 5 cc syringes for flushing NG after gavage feeding
- Several half-gallon milk jugs labeled with different patient names and varied types of high-calorie formulas.
- Refrigerator to store special mix high-calorie formulas. (This can be simulated by utilizing a tabletop with the milk jugs placed on top. An index card can be used to indicate "Formula Refrigerator.")
- Bottles and nipples
- Cup of hot water to warm bottle of formula (which had been stored in refrigerator)
- Water to flush NG after gavage feeding
- Watch or clock to time feeding
- Bedside flow sheet for documentation
- Diapers
- Scale to weigh diapers (To improvise, a designated area outside the patient's room can be labeled as dirty utility room. An index card can have a number recorded to indicate the weight.)
- Pacifier, mobile, tape recorder and lullaby tape all for infant stimulation
- Baby blankets
- Infant seat
- Name band

■ Bedside flow sheet for documentation

Resources needed:

■ Pediatric drug text

■ NG tube policy: Insertion and placement protocols

Simulator level:

■ Static infant manikin or medium-fidelity HPS

Participants: Four people will be needed to run this scenario, including one student nurse, one clinical instructor to observe and prompt through the simulation, one family member (either teen mom or grandmother), and one RT/OT.

Scenario Implementation:

The student first receives report from the clinical instructor, asks questions related to the infant's history or care, and then proceeds into the patient's room. After entering the room, the student should wash hands and make an introduction to the mom/grandmother at the bedside. The student should check the infant's ID band and complete a head-to-toe assessment. Obtaining vital signs, changing the infant's diaper, and cleansing the perineum all should be done following the physical exam. Plan of care for the day should be conveyed to mom/grandmother, and any parental needs should be addressed. The RT will then enter the room and state that the infant is due for an albuterol nebulizer. The student can accept or decline the assistance from the RT. If the student asks the RT to come back, a time must be agreed on. The clinical instructor may prompt the student to utilize this time to document assessment findings or to plan for next steps. The student should review the respiratory plan of care with the RT and confer assessment findings. Once the RT begins the nebulizer treatment, the student should leave the room to weigh the diaper and then prepare a warm bottle of high-calorie formula. When the student returns to the room, the RT will have completed the nebulizer treatment and will be ready to leave. The student should take a moment to reassess breath sounds, check on infant status, and speak with the RT to see how the infant tolerated the treatment. After responding, the RT will exit and the OT will enter the room. The OT will inquire if now is a good time to work with the infant on oral feeding. The student can accept or decline the assistance from the OT. The clinical instructor may encourage the student to utilize this time for documentation and to review the policy of NG tube feedings. After several minutes, the OT will state that the infant has tired and will need the remainder of the formula administered via the NG tube. The student should then proceed to check placement, administer the formula via gavage, flush with water, and secure the tube. Total intake and output should be accurately recorded on the bedside chart, and all documentation should be updated.

Instructor Interventions

The clinical instructor (faculty person) should present a succinct overall report to the student prior to the student entering the patient's room. The early morning needs of the infant (assessment, nebulizer, and feeding) should be emphasized. The instructor should then support the student in decision making and may need to guide the student when collaborating with the RT and OT. The instructor may also prompt the student to see which tasks might be delegated to a nonlicensed professional (nursing assistant) if the tasks are overwhelming. Gentle reminders for good hand washing may be needed throughout the simulation, particularly when leaving and entering the room.

Evaluative Criteria:
Students will be evaluated based on the degree to which they bundle care and with or without coaching perform the actions outlined (Table 16.1).

G. Debriefing Guidelines

The faculty member may choose to debrief with the student participant individually or may choose to review the experience with the entire class.

Questions used for debriefing:

1. How did you feel when you received the initial report from the clinical instructor? Did the history and care overwhelm you for this complex cardiac infant?
2. What was it like for you to interact with a teen mom? Grandmother? Were you anxious to have the parent present while you were interacting with the infant? Was it difficult to address the parent needs (family-centered care) as a part of your plan for the day?
3. What was it like to coordinate care with the RT?
4. Why did you choose to have the RT deliver the nebulizer before feeding the infant? Did the treatment improve ease of breathing, breath sounds, or oxygenation?
5. What is the benefit of administering a nebulizer treatment prior to oral feeding for this cardiac infant?
6. What was it like to coordinate care with the OT? Was this specialist a benefit or hindrance to providing care for your patient?
7. What was the overall impact of bundling morning care for this cardiac infant?
8. When were there opportunities to provide education to the parent? Please describe.
9. What worked well for you in this simulation?
10. What might you have done differently?

H. Suggestions/Key Features to Replicate or Improve

Piloting this scenario with another student prior to the actual run is highly recommended and is helpful in identifying glitches, missing equipment, and timing. Also, having all scenario participants present for the trial is key. Participants who are not able to make the trial run are at a disadvantage and may not fully understand their role, which may change the outcome of the actual simulation. Also, the student participant should be provided the history of the infant and the goals for the day shift in advance so that he or she can prepare for the simulation.

16.1 Evaluating Student Criteria in a Nursing Simulation Scenario

Behavior	Independent	Prompting	Appropriate Order
Washes hands			
Introduces self to parent			
Checks patient's identification band			
Performs head-to-toe assessment			
Assesses vital signs and oxygen saturation			
Performs diaper change, perineal care, and hand washing			
Plan of care reviewed with parent			
Parental needs addressed			
Coordinates care with RT and confers respiratory assessment			
Diaper weighed			
Formula warmed and prepared in bottle with nipple			
Returns to reassess patient's breath sounds and confers with RT regarding effect of nebulizer treatment			
Coordinates care with OT			
Reviews NG tube policy			
Verifies NG tube placement			
Administers NG feeding tube via gavage			
Administers NG tube water flush and tube is secured			
Document assessment, NG tube placement, and I & O			

RT, respiratory therapist; OT, occupational therapist; NG, nasogastric; I & O, input and output.

I. Recommendations for Further Use

The simulation presented focuses on the physiologic needs of a cardiac infant and was adapted from a real-life situation. However, this scenario could be easily altered to focus on psychosocial, financial, spiritual, or health issues related to either the teen mom or the grandmother. This would further highlight the role of the pediatric nurse and the obligation that the nurse has to address the family as partners in care.

In the future, this one case may be divided into parts to form several shorter simulations and could be integrated within the class over the entire semester. Toward the end of the semester, the simulation could then be run in its entirety. For example, an initial simulation may focus on adolescent development, and the student would need to engage in a conversation with the mom and discuss what it is like for the teen to be a new mom with a medically complex infant. A second scenario may focus on medication administration for the infant, and the student would need to demonstrate safe dosage for weight and administration. Another scenario may focus on the student performing NG tube placement and verification. These shorter scenarios would then build confidence and competency for students to put it all together at the end of the semester.

A final recommendation may be to have this one case scenario cross several semesters and several courses. For example, the family in this simulation could be introduced in a medical-surgical course where the grandmother's hypertension and obesity are issues that are specifically addressed. The next semester, the same family may be presented in an obstetrics course where teen pregnancy and prenatal health is the focus. As well, the same case could be reintroduced in a pediatric course, in which the focus would be an infant who is born with a congenital heart defect.

J. Discussion of Simulation-Based Pedagogy and How This New Technology Has Contributed to Improved Student Outcomes

This was the first time that this simulation was run in an undergraduate pediatric nursing course. Students in the larger classroom were able to view the simulation via a live video; however, sound delivery was inconsistent at times. The group as a whole described the learning as valuable, because in reality, not all of them will be able to experience caring for an infant with congenital heart disease. This experience gave them a glimpse as to what the care may entail. The main participant stated that it was particularly helpful to practice this inclusive care even though one may stumble or not get it right. The student believed it was better to experience it once than not at all, especially before performing on a real-life patient. Additionally, this one participant supported the idea of standardized patients and simulations in every nursing class to really enhance learning!

The above student comments are supported by an increasing number of articles in the nursing literature. Research conducted by Ham and O'Rourke (2004) found that students experience an easier transition into their first clinical setting once having participated in simulation activity. Developing competency in nursing care takes practice in a variety of health care settings and with a diverse sample of patients and families. In the majority of the nursing programs today, no two students will have the exact clinical experience. As faculty, we cannot guarantee similar learning in the clinical setting. However, with clinical simulations, it may be possible for many students to have similar learning outcomes if they are provided the same opportunities (Larew, Lessans, Spunt, Foster, & Covington, 2006).

References

American Association of Colleges of Nursing. (2007). *The October 22, 2007 draft revision of the essentials of baccalaureate education for professional nursing practice.* Washington, DC: AACN.

Ball, J., & Bindler, R. (2008). *Pediatric nursing: Caring for children* (4th ed.). Upper Saddle River, NJ: Pearson Education.

Ham, K., & O'Rourke, E. (2004). Clinical preparation for beginning nursing students: An experiential learning activity. *Nurse Educator, 29,* 139–141.

Hockenberry, M., & Wilson, D. (2007). *Wong's nursing care of infants and children* (8th ed.). St Louis, MO: Mosby.

Huffman, S., Jarczyk, K., O'Brien, E., Pieper, P., & Bayne, A. (2004). Methods to confirm feeding tube placement: Application of research in practice. *Pediatric Nursing, 30,* 10–13.

Larew, C., Lessans, S., Spunt, D., Foster, D., & Covington, B. (2006). Innovations in clinical simulation: Application of Benner's theory in an interactive patient care simulation. *Nursing Education Perspectives, 27,* 6–21.

Oermann, M., & Gaberson, K. (2006). *Evaluation and testing in nursing education* (2nd ed.). New York: Springer.

Verger, J. T., & Lebet, R. (Eds.). (2008). *AACN: Procedure manual for pediatric acute and critical care.* St. Louis, MO: Saunders.

Westhus, N. (2004). Methods to test feeding tube placement in children. *MCN, the American Journal of Maternal Child Nursing, 29,* 282–291.

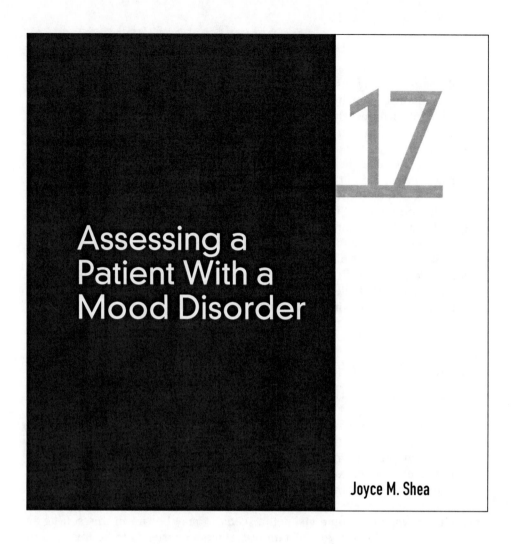

17

Assessing a Patient With a Mood Disorder

Joyce M. Shea

This chapter presents a simulation activity that incorporates student knowledge of psychiatric illness and risk assessment with a focus on mood disorders and substance abuse. The simulation exercise builds on skills in therapeutic communication, lethality assessment, and recognition of signs and symptoms of major depression and alcohol abuse. Postscenario discussion can assist in clarifying issues in documentation, patient rights, and legal requirements of mental health nursing practice.

A. Discussion of Implementation of Simulation-Based Pedagogy in Each Contributor's Individualized Teaching

Faculty in baccalaureate nursing programs face many difficulties in their efforts to connect theory to practice for students. In a mental health nursing course, the difficulties can be compounded by the abstract nature of the content and the students' potential discomfort with the unique processes associated with mental health nursing care. Taking a broad-based approach to simulation allows the mental health nursing instructor to incorporate a variety of highly interactive strategies, many of which have traditionally been used to set the stage for the students' entrance into clinical sites. For example, I have frequently relied on role-play exercises to sharpen communication techniques and build confidence in students as they prepare for their initial exposure to acute-care psychiatric patients. Creative use of case studies has also provided a means for students to demonstrate their skill at comprehensive and interdisciplinary care planning. Because mental health nursing students need to integrate multiple sources of information on a patient, including observations on affect (e.g., facial expression) and speech (e.g., tone, rate, patterns, etc.), the creation of a high-fidelity simulation using a human patient simulator (HPS) may not be the most effective teaching strategy. The following scenario has been created for use with a standardized patient (SP)—a human actor, paid or volunteer—who brings the situation to life and challenges the students to draw on diverse areas of theoretical knowledge as the interaction progresses. Students can also be assigned auxiliary roles, such as family member, employer, or roommate.

B. Description of Educational Materials Available in Your Teaching Area and Relative to Your Specialty

The scenario can be run in a number of settings and requires minimal prep or set up. At the Fairfield University School of Nursing (FUSON) Robin Kanarek Learning Resource Center, there is a home health area designed for simulations in mental health or community/public health care. Accessories include a twin bed, a table with lamp, an upholstered chair, a throw rug, a floor lamp, and a phone. If students in the Mental Health Nursing course have the opportunity to conduct psychiatric home visits, the scenario may be run in this setting as a mobile outreach, with roles for family members or friends to be involved in the interaction. Otherwise, the scenario may be run as an interaction in an employee health clinic, a walk-in clinic, or an urgent care section of the Emergency Department (ED). The setting for these requires either two chairs and a desk or an exam table and a chair or stool for the nurse conducting the assessment interview. Blood pressure cuffs, a Breathalyzer machine, and a "clinic" phone should be available. Intake forms (including mental health assessment), depression screening forms, and substance abuse screening forms should also be present.

C. Specific Objective for Simulation Utilization Within a Specific Course and the Overall Program

The main objective of the scenario is accurate assessment of psychiatric symptoms and risk factors for self-harm. The nursing process is used to identify priorities among patient needs, and an evidence-based plan of care is established. Students at FUSON who are taking Mental Health Nursing are in the first semester of the third year of their baccalaureate program, having completed one prior clinical course in Geriatric Nursing, a lab course in Health

Assessment, and core science courses in Chemistry, Anatomy and Physiology, Microbiology, and Developmental Psychology. Concurrently with Mental Health Nursing, they take their first Medical Nursing course and a theory course in Pathopharmacology. They are beginning to work on the integration of content across courses, particularly in the areas of communication and health assessment. The simulation activity presented in this chapter will specifically help students to meet objectives for the Mental Health Nursing course in the following areas: identifying risk factors for psychiatric disorders, developing therapeutic communication skills and planning appropriate evidence-based care for psychiatric patients, recognizing ethical and legal issues as they present in patients with psychiatric illness, and understanding the role of the nurse based on the American Nurses Association's *Standards of Practice for Psychiatric-Mental Health Nursing* (2007).

D. Introduction of Scenario to Include Setting the Scene, Technology Used, Objectives, and Description of Participants

A human actor plays a 28-year-old female who presents to the Employee Health Clinic with complaints of a migraine headache and fatigue. The nursing students are responsible for conducting the initial intake and assessment. They are given the standard forms used for routine clinic visits and are told that they may also make use of any other equipment present in the exam room. The students' goal is to complete an initial assessment and establish a plan of care based on the data collected within 15 minutes. They will be evaluated on their skills in conducting the interview, their ability to gather necessary information and to determine the priority of needs at this time, their appropriate use of equipment and supplies, and the establishment of a comprehensive plan of care for the patient. Additional roles for students may include a coworker or supervisor, family member, or friend.

E. Describe Running of the Scenario

Prior to running the scenario, the human actor playing the SP was given details about the patient's background, including medical and psychiatric history, work and school history, current stressors, and behavioral patterns. She was instructed to provide minimal information until prompted by the student. There was no past medical record available. Students were given access to a phone to allow for contact with other health care providers (e.g., mental health care crisis workers) or a hospital ED as needed. In addition, students could use their personal digital assistants (PDAs) to access information on evidence-based practice related to depression and substance abuse. Although they were unable to access or communicate with the instructor or other students during the scenario, they were given the opportunity to identify additional sources of information they would have liked to use on completion of the interview (e.g., family members).

F. Presentation of Completed Template

Scenario Title: Assessing a Patient With a Mood Disorder (for first-semester, junior-year baccalaureate students in Nursing 305, Mental Health Nursing)

Focus Area:
Psychiatric-Mental Health Nursing, Health Assessment, Risk Assessment

Scenario Description:
Tina Hall is a 28-year-old, single, black female who comes to the Employee Health Clinic complaining of a migraine headache and fatigue. She has been an employee in the Information Technology Department for the past 6 years, having started immediately after graduating with honors from college. She is currently working as interim department manager while her supervisor is out on medical leave. She lives alone in her own apartment and recently became engaged. Although she has experienced migraines on occasion in the past, they are now happening more frequently (1–2 per week) and are becoming more severe (7/10 self-report of pain accompanied by nausea and light sensitivity). She has been feeling extremely stressed and fears being unable to cope with the responsibilities of her job. She has had several recent conflicts with the employees under her supervision. She is having increasing trouble sleeping and has recently begun to have 2 or 3 glasses of wine before going to bed every night. She feels edgy and distressed and wants to be given "something like Ativan" to help calm her nerves and get her through the day. She has no other medical problems and no known allergies.

Scenario Objectives:
Students who successfully complete this scenario exercise will have demonstrated their ability to (1) communicate effectively with a distraught client, (2) recognize the signs and symptoms related to a mood disorder, (3) conduct a substance abuse assessment on the client (see appendices A–B for assessment scales), (4) conduct a lethality assessment (http://www.mh.state.oh.us/cmtymh/soqic/forms/pdf/sq06070.pdf) and (5) offer some appropriate nonpharmacologic interventions to reduce the client's level of stress.

    Successful completion of the simulation activity would also allow the student to meet several of the revised American Association of Colleges of Nursing (2007) *Essentials of Baccalaureate Education for Professional Nursing Practice,* including Essentials I, II, III, VI, and VIII. Areas of the 2007 National Council Licensure Examination for Registered Nurses (NCLEX-RN) test plan categories (NCSBN, 2007) that are covered in the exercise include the following:

    Safe and Effective Care Environment
        Management of Care
            Client Rights
            Establishing Priorities
            Legal Rights and Responsibilities
    Health Promotion and Maintenance
        Health Screening
        High Risk Behaviors

Psychosocial Integrity
Chemical and Other Dependencies
Coping Mechanisms
Crisis Intervention
Grief and Loss
Mental Health Concepts
Psychopathology
Situational Role Changes
Stress Management
Support Systems
Therapeutic Communications
Physiological Integrity
Basic Care and Comfort
Nonpharmacological Comfort Interventions
Rest and Sleep

Setting the Scene:

Equipment needed: Exam table, chair or stool for nurse, blood pressure cuff, Breathalyzer machine, phone, intake and assessment forms, and patient information brochures on anxiety and depression. Students were informed that they would be allowed to use a PDA to access information on evidence-based practice related to treatment of depression and associated risk factors such as suicide (American Psychiatric Association, 2003; National Institute of Mental Health, 2008; University of Michigan Health System, 2005). The SP and the student are the only required participants, but additional roles may be developed for a coworker, family member, or friend.

Scenario Implementation:

The SP was instructed to present with a moderate level of agitation and to focus on physical complaints and her sense of being overwhelmed. All other information would only be divulged in response to student questions. Students were required to respond appropriately to the level of agitation displayed by the SP, utilize effective communication techniques, conduct a thorough health history (physical as well as psychological), perform a lethality assessment and alcohol abuse assessment to determine priorities for care, and implement a short-term plan of action to meet identified needs. The instructor facilitated the student learning through the debriefing process on completion of the scenario.

Evaluation Criteria:

Students were evaluated based on their effective integration of theory with practice (i.e., their ability to elicit the necessary information, gain a thorough understanding of the client's needs, determine the priorities for care, and establish a reasonable plan based on clinical evidence). Their ability to conceptualize the main issues was captured in their efforts to present a plan of care to the client.

Checklist of interventions and assessments:

_____ Introduce self.
_____ Establish therapeutic relationship with patient.

_____ Demonstrate therapeutic communication skills.
_____ Utilize skills to reduce patient agitation.
_____ Obtain information on chief complaint.
_____ Obtain information on past medical history.
_____ Conduct mental status assessment.
_____ Evaluate symptoms of depression.
_____ Conduct lethality assessment.
_____ Evaluate pattern of substance use.
_____ Present patient with nonpharmacologic alternative for stress reduction.
_____ Establish appropriate plan of care with patient.

G. Debriefing Guidelines

At least 15 minutes should be allowed for debriefing and discussion. The instructor may choose to debrief the students individually at first, asking them to reflect on the following questions:

1. Did you prepare for this scenario in any way? If so, how?
2. How would you evaluate your actions throughout the scenario?
3. What actions might you have taken to increase your effectiveness?
4. Was there any issue that arose to which you felt unable to respond?
5. How did this interaction compare with other patient interactions you've experienced?

The following questions may be posed to the larger class:

1. What specific communication techniques were used?
2. What additional areas of assessment needed to be addressed?
3. What additional patient needs could be identified?
4. What would you do if the patient indicated that she was intending to commit suicide?
5. What information should/must be included in the employee health record?
6. How much information can or should be shared in a referral for mental health care?
7. In what ways has your understanding of the role of the baccalaureate-prepared nurse increased?

H. Suggestions/Key Features to Replicate or Improve

The key features of communication and assessment can be replicated in scenarios with patients who have various diagnoses, ages, comorbidities, and risk factors. The scenario, as is, can only be implemented if students have completed background reading on stress, mood disorders, suicidality, substance abuse, and therapeutic communication. In addition, students will benefit from having completed the first several weeks of mental health clinical prior to attempting the scenario.

I. Recommendations for Further Use

This simulation could be developed with a focus on an elderly client in the home setting or a crisis situation in the community. Additional legal and ethical issues, such as competency and involuntary hospitalization, could be introduced. The simulation activity described here can easily be modified for graduate psychiatric NP students by having the student play the role of an outpatient clinician who is performing an intake assessment and requiring them to develop a plan of care that includes pharmacologic as well as cognitive-behavioral interventions.

J. Discussion of Simulation-Based Pedagogy and How This New Technology Has Contributed to Improved Student Outcomes

A simulation-based pedagogy may seem initially to have limited usefulness in a mental health nursing class, but the impact could at least equal that achieved in any other class if approached in the right way. Case studies and role-play have long been deemed appropriate methods to help bridge the gap between theory and practice for baccalaureate students. Use of an SP and integration of a well-designed scenario could lead to tremendous opportunities for significant learning to take place. Students are more likely to be active participants if the class activity is interesting to them, and the debriefing period will allow for a sharing of thoughts and reactions that makes the learning process personal and memorable. The student who takes on the main role in the scenario will have a solid experience on which to build his or her understanding of psychiatric assessment, suicide risk, substance abuse, and stress response and reduction. Basing the scenario in a location other than an inpatient psychiatric unit will also promote a greater understanding of the application of mental health nursing principles across settings.

Appendix A: CAGE Questionnaire

Purpose: The purpose of the CAGE Questionnaire is to detect alcoholism.

Clinical utility: The CAGE Questionnaire is a very useful bedside, clinical desk instrument and has become the favorite of many family practice and general internists—also very popular in nursing.

Groups with whom this instrument has been used: Adults and adolescents (over 16 years)

Format: Very brief, relatively nonconfrontational questionnaire for detection of alcoholism, usually directed "have you ever" but may be focused to delineate past or present

Administration time: Less than 1 minute

Scoring time: Instantaneous

Computer scoring? No

Administrator training and qualifications: No training required for administration; it is easy to learn, easy to remember, and easy to replicate.

Fee for use: No

Available from: May be downloaded from the Project Cork Web site: http://www.projectcork.org

Scoring: One point for each positive answer.
Score of 1–3 should create a high index of suspicion and warrants further evaluation.

Score of 1	80% are alcohol dependent
Score of 2	89% are alcohol dependent
Score of 3	99% are alcohol dependent
Score of 4	100% are alcohol dependent

CAGE

Name _____

Date _____

Score _____

	Yes	No
1. Have you ever felt you should **C**ut down on your drinking ?	1	—
2. Have people **A**nnoyed you by criticizing your drinking?	1	—
3. Have you ever felt bad or **G**uilty about your drinking?	1	—
4. Have you had an **E**ye opener first thing in the morning to steady nerves or get rid of a hangover?	1	—

Source: Ewing, J. A. (1984). Detecting alcoholism, the CAGE questionnaire. *Journal of the American Medical Association, 252,* 1905–1907. From Health Services/ Information Technology Text, National Library of Medicine, Retrieved June 12, 2008, from http://www.ncbi.nlm.nih.gov/books/bv.fcgi?rid=hstat5.section. 77081

Appendix B: Zung Self-Rating Depression Scale

Patient's Initials _____

Date of Assessment _____

Please read each statement and decide how much of the time the statement describes how you have been feeling during the past several days.

Make check mark (√) in appropriate column.	A little of the time	Some of the time	Good part of the time	Most of the time
1. I feel down-hearted and blue				
2. Morning is when I feel the best				
3. I have crying spells or feel like it				
4. I have trouble sleeping at night				
5. I eat as much as I used to				
6. I still enjoy sex				
7. I notice that I am losing weight				
8. I have trouble with constipation				
9. My heart beats faster than usual				
10. I get tired for no reason				
11. My mind is as clear as it used to be				
12. I find it easy to do the things I used to				
13. I am restless and can't keep still				
14. I feel hopeful about the future				
15. I am more irritable than usual				
16. I find it easy to make decisions				
17. I feel that I am useful and needed				
18. My life is pretty full				
19. I feel that others would be better off if I were dead				
20. I still enjoy the things I used to do				

Source: Adapted from Zung, W. W. K. (1965). A self-rating depression scale. *Archives of General Psychiatry, 12,* 63–70. From: Department of Psychiatry, University of Massachusetts.

KEY TO SCORING THE ZUNG SELF-RATING DEPRESSION SCALE Consult this key for the value (1–4) that correlates with patients' responses to each statement. Add up the numbers for a total score. Most people with depression score between 50 and 69. The highest possible score is 80.

Make check mark (√) in appropriate column.	A little of the time	Some of the time	Good part of the time	Most of the time
1. I feel down-hearted and blue	1	2	3	4
2. Morning is when I feel the best	4	3	2	1
3. I have crying spells or feel like it	1	2	3	4
4. I have trouble sleeping at night	1	2	3	4
5. I eat as much as I used to	4	3	2	1
6. I still enjoy sex	4	3	2	1
7. I notice that I am losing weight	1	2	3	4
8. I have trouble with constipation	1	2	3	4
9. My heart beats faster than usual	1	2	3	4
10. I get tired for no reason	1	2	3	4
11. My mind is as clear as it used to be	4	3	2	1
12. I find it easy to do the things I used to	4	3	2	1
13. I am restless and can't keep still	1	2	3	4
14. I feel hopeful about the future	4	3	2	1
15. I am more irritable than usual	1	2	3	4
16. I find it easy to make decisions	4	3	2	1
17. I feel that I am useful and needed	4	3	2	1
18. My life is pretty full	4	3	2	1
19. I feel that others would be better off if I were dead	1	2	3	4
20. I still enjoy the things I used to do	4	3	2	1

Medical School. (2008). Retrieved June 12, 2008, from http://healthnet.umassmed. edu/mhealth/mhscales.cfm

References

American Association of Colleges of Nursing. (2007). *The October 22, 2007 draft revision of the essentials of baccalaureate education for professional nursing practice.* Washington, DC: AACN.

American Nurses Association. (2007). *Psychiatric-mental health nursing: Scope and standards of practice.* Silver Spring, MD: nursesbooks.org

American Psychiatric Association. (2003). *Practice guideline for the assessment and treatment of patients with suicidal behaviors.* Retrieved February 19, 2008, from http://www.guideline. gov/summary/summary.aspx?ss=15&doc_id=4529&string=%22practice+guideline+for+ the+assessment%22+and+%22treatment+of+patients+with+suicidal+behaviors%22

National Council of State Boards of Nursing. (2007). *NCLEX-RN examination: Test plan for the National Council Licensure Examination for Registered Nurses.* Retrieved June 12, 2008, from https://www.ncsbn.org/RN_Test_Plan_2007_Web.pdf

National Institute of Mental Health. (2008). *What are the symptoms of depression?* Retrieved February 19, 2008, from http://www.nimh.nih.gov/health/publications/depression/ symptoms.shtml

University of Michigan Health System. (2005). *Depression.* Retrieved February 19, 2008, from http://www.guideline.gov/summary/summary.aspx?ss=15&doc_id=8330&string= depression

18

Communication With an Elderly Client

**Lilian Rafeldt,
Heather Bader, and
Suzanne Turner**

A. Discussion of Implementation of Simulation-Based Pedagogy in Each Contributor's Individualized Teaching

Simulation has been used at Three Rivers Community College throughout the curriculum for many years. Role-play within the Helene Fuld Nursing Laboratory simulating patient care environments has assisted students with multiple learning styles to master content and perform proficiently within the clinical setting. Faculty strives to address aural, visual, and kinesthetic learning styles while fostering critical thinking within the discipline of nursing. Critical thinking is a practice rather than a doctrine that helps the student to draw correct conclusions within a nursing environment. It is easy to carry out rote procedures rather than assessing and "thinking out" what to do in a situation. When students learn how to use broad concepts, they can perform procedures long after graduation (Nosich, 2008). In recent years, static and high-fidelity manikins have become the patient.

In preparation for the nursing laboratory at the New Three Rivers Community College unification site, the nursing director, Linda Perfetto, the laboratory staff, Heather Bader and Sue Turner, and faculty, Teri Ashton, Judy

Snayd, Mary Browning, and Lili Rafeldt, collaborated with the Information Technology Department members and consultants to develop a program and environment conducive to high-fidelity simulation. Multiple strategies were employed to develop case scenarios, including site visits to established simulation labs, education, Web sites to share cases, and graduate students developing simulation scenarios for curriculum development and credit toward their degree. Laboratory staff held a contest where students named the human patient simulator (HPS). Targeted faculty and laboratory staff continue to facilitate statewide initiatives promoting growth within the Connecticut Community College Nursing Program, state, and nation. This multifaceted approach in creation of laboratory class work, independent study material, and theory presentation content has encouraged growth without depleting resources or taxing staff.

B. Description of Educational Materials Available in Your Teaching Area and Relative to Your Specialty

Some of the first successful simulation experiences included students who demonstrated critical thinking ability while caring for clients with orthopedic conditions. After completing the learning unit, students signed up in groups of three to four to care for Mr. Bilirubin, who had a right total hip replacement. He had one of eight complications; the students had to identify the complication correctly and then implement appropriate care. As there were eight possible complications, students could not listen to "the grapevine" to prepare their actual care. Critical thinking skills within the moment in the discipline of nursing were required. Students rated this experience as an extremely positive activity. The simulation was conceived by a faculty member, designed in conjunction with laboratory staff, delivered by laboratory staff, and evaluated via a report prepared by the group and submitted to the faculty member. Laboratory staff conducted a debriefing session and gave immediate feedback. Collaboration and use of each other's strengths promoted success in development, implementation, and evaluation.

Another successful simulation experience included students who were returning or transferring into the program at varying levels. Simulation exercises were constructed to include outcomes from previous program levels. Students completed the simulations with laboratory staff, debriefed, and were evaluated by faculty for entering course placements. Simulation was not the only criteria for placement levels.

Program development was one component in fostering growth of simulation at Three Rivers Community College. New classroom spaces were also designed to include simulation areas and control rooms with debriefing areas. Wiring, cameras, and network ability allows for broadcasts to lecture classrooms as well as seminar areas. Three SimMen®, SimBaby®, Nurse Anne Vital Sim®, and Patient Kelly Vital Sim® begin the complement of simulators from Laerdal. Some beds have been left empty to encourage active learning in other formats, but wiring is in place for continued growth in high-fidelity simulation.

Simulation in nursing education provides a foundation for knowledge, skill performance, collaboration, critical thinking, and self-confidence development. In this simulation scenario, Communication With an Elderly Client, students will have the opportunity to reinforce previously learned content and explore principles used in communication with the older adult. Leo Vygotsky (1978) defined *scaffolding* as an instruction technique. The scaffolds facilitate a student's ability to build on prior knowledge and internalize new information. This technique enriches the following scenario.

C. Specific Objective for Simulation Utilization Within a Specific Course and the Overall Program

Nurses assess, interview, examine, and gather data to develop plans and implement and evaluate care. Nurses of the 21st century will use critical thinking when communicating with elders—the most rapidly expanding group of the population. Development of expert skills in communication facilitates efficient client-centered care, resolution of illness, and promotion of health. This scenario will focus on communication with an elderly client in the hospital. A generalist nurse provides direct and indirect care.

The scenario can be used in an Introduction to Nursing or Gerontologic Nursing course or as a tutoring tool for students who desire reinforcement of learning to support clinical practice. It may be used as an individual or group exercise. This scenario builds on previous learning, utilizing principles of scaffolding described by Vygotsky (1978), while focusing on achievement of new outcomes. "Standard nursing behaviors when interacting with a client" are expected in each scenario; new outcomes are added. The scenario can be enhanced in advanced nursing courses when the client becomes deaf, aphasic, or visually impaired or is diagnosed with dementia. The scenario can be extended to develop nursing diagnoses and plans of care.

D. Introduction of Scenario to Include Setting the Scene, Technology Used, Objectives, and Description of Participants

Students will enter a "Nursing Lab Hospital." Evaluators can predetermine whether a uniform or any other equipment from home is required to care for the client. At the bedside, the student or students will find Mrs. Bilirubin, as described in the scenario description below. Choices are provided for high-fidelity or live role-play scenarios. Consider 20 students entering the lab: 5 students could be assigned to act as the "active scenario participants," while the other 15 students could be assigned to be observers using the evaluative checklists. The student observers could watch the scenario within the same room or in an observation classroom, depending on the constructed environment. Principles of teamwork can be fostered. As multiple simulations are required throughout a semester, roles can be rotated.

E. Describe Running of the Scenario

Frames within high-fidelity simulation can be used to assist progression of the simulation. Student actions can drive progression toward new frames, or check boxes completed by the controller can be used. The controller would identify "done," "not done," or "done with prompt" within the program. The use of evaluative checklists by multiple observers encourages assessment, reflection, and professional growth for all participating in the process. Complexity in feedback and active learning can be embraced by utilizing evaluative checklists for primary objectives as well as for standard nursing behaviors when interacting with a client.

F. Presentation of Completed Template

Title: Communication With an Elderly Client

Focus Area:
First year of Nursing or Gerontology Course

Scenario Description:
An 85-year-old woman is admitted to a medical-surgical unit with a suspected urinary tract infection. She is a widow of 3 years, was married for 62 years, has three adult children, and lives in her own home with an unmarried son. She has a history of two incidents of congestive heart failure (CHF) 4 years ago, a total hysterectomy 22 years ago, a left total knee replacement (LTK) 15 years ago, and situational depression when her husband passed away. The "nurse" or participant in this scenario will practice principles of communication with the elderly woman.

The woman presents with the following vital signs—BP: 140/88, P: 90, RR: 22, and T: 99F. She complains of (c/o) falling into her chair at home, dribbling when trying to get to the bathroom, fatigue, and not being hungry for 1 week. Her physician evaluated a urinalysis and CBC with differential and recommended admission to the hospital for further evaluation and treatment. She is 5′5″ tall and weighs 160 pounds.

The scenario starts with the "nurse" entering the room.

Learning Method:
Active learning within the cognitive, psychomotor, and affective domains through high-fidelity simulator, role-play, or case study.

Primary Learning Outcomes:
During and after completing the simulation experience, the student will be able to do the following:

1. Identify intrinsic and extrinsic factors that affect communication with an elderly client.
2. Identify, perform, and discuss strategies that can increase communication with an elderly client.
3. Identify client conditions that can contribute to impaired communication.
4. Perform and discuss therapeutic communication skills in phases of the nurse–client relationship.

5. Discuss how attitudes affect behavior and propose changes that could be made in future interactions with elderly clients.

The National Council of State Boards of Nursing National Council Licensure Examination for Registered Nurses (NCLEX-RN) test plan categories and subcategories (NCSBN, 2007) included in this scenario are as follows:

Safe and Effective Care Environment
    Management of Care
        Client Rights
    Safety and Infection Control
        Safe Use of Equipment
Health Promotion and Maintenance
        Aging Process
Psychosocial Integrity
        Therapeutic Communications
Physiological Integrity
    Basic Care and Comfort
        Elimination
        Personal Hygiene
    Pharmacological and Parenteral Therapies
        Dosage Calculation
        Medication Administration
        Parenteral/Intravenous Therapies
    Reduction of Risk Potential
        Potential for Complications from Surgical Procedures and Health Alterations
        Vital Signs
    Physiological Adaptation
        Illness Management

Student Preparation for the Simulation:

Required readings: Required readings relate to communication and the elderly in your curriculum. Chapters from a Fundamentals in Nursing or Gerontologic text or a journal article would be listed.

Web sites to explore:
    John A. Hartford Foundation, http://www.jhartfound.org/index.htm
    Building Academic Geriatric Nursing Capacity, http://www.geriatricnursing.org/

Completed medication sheet/card: Information sheet/card for cefazolin (Ancef) 1 g IV; nystatin (Mycostatin) 400,000 U po; furosemide (Lasix) 60 mg po; potassium supplement (K-Dur) 40 meqs po; digoxin (Lanoxin) 0.25 mg po

Review of standard nursing behaviors when interacting with a client: Verification of client orders and plan of care, identification of client, introduction of self and explanation of reason there, asepsis as appropriate, preparation and gathering of equipment/supplies needed, maintenance of privacy and HIPAA standards, appropriate ergonomic/body mechanics when assessing or performing care, maintenance of a safe environment (bed position, call bell, and equipment placement), and documentation. Use of the evaluative criteria for standard nursing behaviors when interacting with a client (as shown later in this chapter) succinctly identifies the behaviors.

Completion of survey: Beliefs about the elderly—answer the following questions with a yes or no. Bring this to the simulation. Highlights will be discussed in debriefing.

1. Most old people are sick.
2. Most old people are in nursing homes.
3. Most old people are retired.
4. Most old people would like to live in a warm climate.
5. Most old people live in poverty.
6. Most old people cannot learn as easily as when they were young.
7. Most old people are hard of hearing.
8. Most old people have no interest in sex.
9. Most old people are more religious than young people.

Setting the Scene:

1. Female wig on head
2. Peripheral IV in left arm (nondominant)—IV catheter, tape, ordered intravenous fluid on infusion pump
3. Female genitalia
4. Sequential compression devices, bilaterally on lower extremities
5. Equipment to measure vital signs (thermometer, stethoscope, sphygmomanometer)
6. Hospital gown
7. ID bracelet with name, age, physician, medical record number, and allergies
8. Collection container for routine urinalysis and culture and sensitivity
9. Curtain or ability to create private assessment area
10. Available oxygen via nasal cannula tubing
11. Medication administration tools: drug handbook or personal digital assistant with med program, measuring cup, IVPB tubing, simulated ordered meds, water pitcher with glass
12. Client medical record that includes orders, history and physical, medication administration record (MAR), intake and output record (I & O), and progress documentation forms.
13. Telephone (for access to admitting nurse and physician)

Participants needed:

1. Transfer assistant (if needed)
2. Lab member (if role-play used)
3. Voice of admitting nurse (can be simulation controller, other student, or Preprogrammed Handler)
4. Voice of physician (can be simulation controller, other student, or Preprogrammed Handler)
5. Simulation controller (if high-fidelity HPS used)
6. Mrs. Bilirubin (other prepped student nurse)
7. Observers to participate in debriefing (if used as a group exercise)

Scenario Implementation:

Expected run time is 15 to 20 minutes. The "nurse" is given a report from the admitting nurse via the telephone as the client is transported to the unit via stretcher. The medical record is brought to the unit with the client. Another student can assist with transfer, or this step can be eliminated by having the client in the bed to begin the scenario.

The report given is as follows: Mrs. Bilirubin, age 85. Vital signs: BP: 140/88, P: 90, RR: 22, T: 99. She complained of falling into her chair at home, dribbling when trying to get to the bathroom, being tired, and not being hungry for a week. Dr. Smith evaluated a urinalysis and CBC with differential and recommended admission to rule out sepsis and urinary tract infection. Mrs. Bilirubin also has a fungal infection within her mouth. She is 5'5" tall and weighs 160 pounds.

Mrs. Bilirubin is a widow of 3 years, was married for 62 years, has three adult children, and lives in her own home with an unmarried son. She has a history of two incidents of CHF 4 years ago, a hysterectomy 22 years ago, an LTK replacement 15 years ago, and situational depression when her husband passed away.

Physician/provider orders include the following:

Admit to 1 South
Activity level: Bed rest today
Diet: Low NA, low cholesterol
D5 ½ NS at 100 cc per hour
UA and urine C/S
Cefazolin 1 g iv stat
SCDs
V/S q 4 h
Oxygen 2 L via nasal cannula titrated to maintain and PaO_2 of 92% prn
Lasix 40 mg po qd
KDur tab 40 meqs po qd
Digoxin 0.250 mg po qd
Mycostatin 400,000 U qid swish ½ of dose in each side of mouth; hold
Tylenol 650 mg po q 4 h prn for T above 101

The student begins the scenario by transferring Mrs. Bilirubin from the stretcher to the bed and assessing the patient. The student will be expected to focus on primary learning outcomes; however, basic principles of safety and infection control nurse–client behaviors will also be expected.

Three frames are constructed within a high-simulation program. Frame 1 lasts 5 minutes, frame 2 lasts 10 minutes, and frame 3 only occurs if interventions are not done within frames 1 and 2. A microphone can be used during the exercise, or voice handlers can be built into the scenario. Table 18.1 shows the scenario for a high-simulation program (such as SimMan® by Laerdal) but can be adapted for roleplay.

The simulation controller concludes the scenario and allows the students (and observers of group exercise) to reflect on behaviors within the scenario for 5 to 10 minutes. A 12-item Communication in the Elderly true-false quiz is given and will be self-evaluated by the student(s) in the debriefing.

Scenario Progression Outline

Timing	Mrs. Bilirubin	Expected Actions	Prompts, Questions, Teaching Points	Other Prompts/Cues
Frame 1: First 5 minutes	Temp: 99 A: Sinus tach: 90 BP: 140/88 Monitor controls: SpO$_2$: 98% RR: 22 Auscultation sounds: Lungs: Clear Heart: S1S2 Bowel: Normative	Verify orders. Wash hands. Introduce self: face client, use normal tone. Turn lights on.	Is environment conducive for interview—light, background noise, private, warm? Is student speaking face to face with the client; not off to the side, hands away from your face, not chewing gum?	Understanding that presentation of disease in an elderly client may be atypical; falls may indicate infection.
Can go to 3rd frame if client not acknowledged or no appropriate response to patient's complaint of pain given.	Use microphone or put in program as handlers (SimMan): "My name is Mrs. Bilirubin. I'm here to feel better. I've been tired and wetting myself. It is so embarrassing. I never wet myself."	Identify client by ID band and ask client name, where she is, and why. Provide privacy for client in semi-fowler position. Identify IVF and site; assess match to order. Assess and document V/S.	Is the student speaking in a normal way; not shouting? Is time given for conversation? Did student use three-item recall screening technique? Needed? No cognitive impairments seen. Does student acknowledge client's suffering? Does student use open-ended questions when gathering information?	A temperature of 99 may indicate a fever in an elderly client. Incontinence is abnormal in the normal aging process.
	Whispering. "I'm sorry I'm here. I'm not sure what will happen to me. My mouth hurts."	Answer client questions. Determine that pain may interfere with assessment and that an intervention is available.	Does student's nonverbal and verbal convey a sense of caring? Does student recognize pain may interfere with communication?	
Frame 2: Next 10 minutes 6–15 minutes	A: Sinus tach: 100 BP: 140/90 Monitor controls: SpO$_2$: 96% RR: 24	Validate cefazolin and mycostatin order; prepare and administer using safe medication practices.	Does student explain medications to client and validate understanding?	Reinforcement of previous learning—safe medication administration.

	Auscultation sounds: Lungs: Clear Heart: S1S2 Bowel: Normative		This represents scaffolding or building on previous learning to increase the complex dimensions of a student.
Can go to 3rd frame if no action taken in response to client not understanding instructions or stating she is wet.	Using microphone or put in program as handlers (SimMan®): "My name is Mrs. Bilirubin. I was born on March 7th." "What do you want me to do with that medicine? Did you say ish is outh?"	Document: Explains procedure. places bed in high position. collects urine specimens. Returns bed to lowest position.	Does student enunciate instructions clearly: "Swish this around your mouth"? Consonants are not heard as well. Is the student using a low-pitch voice? High-pitch sounds are the first sounds an elderly client may not hear.
	"Some of the urine wet my bed. I don't want to talk anymore."	Label, and place in bag for delivery to lab.	Does the student change linen. providing comfort to the client before continuing the assessment?
	"Thank you. I feel better. I'm tired. Can you come back later?"	Clean client. remove wet underpad. and replace with dry pad. Wash hands.	Does the student complete the assessment or let the client sleep? What is the rationale given by student?
Frame 3: Occurs if no nursing intervention for pain. lack of understanding by nurse. or client is left wet.	Temp: 99.8 A: Sinus tach: 130 BP: 150/98 Monitor controls: SpO2: 92% RR: 28 Auscultation sounds: Lungs: Clear Heart: S1S2 Bowel: Normative	Recognize intervention was required.	Does student identify that client may exhibit distress when communication is not effective?
	Using microphone or put in program as handlers (SimMan®): Moaning. "This is horrible. Help me."		

BP. blood pressure: SpO2. oxygen saturation: RR. respiratory rate: IVF. intravenous fluids: V/S. vital signs.

18.2	Evaluative Criteria for Standard Nursing Behaviors When Interacting With a Client		
Behavior	Independent	Prompt	Comments
Verify orders			
Turn lights on; assess/intervene for safe environment			
Introduce self/role			
Wash hands			
Identify client by identification band and verbal method			
Position ergonomically/provide privacy			
Identify IVF, site health; assess match to order			
Assess/document V/S			
Notify provider if needed			
Address pain			
Answer questions			
Perform interventions appropriately			
Complete other assessments/interventions			
Document			

IVF, intravenous fluids; V/S, vital signs.

Evaluative Criteria for Standard Nursing Behaviors When Interacting With a Client:
Students will be given feedback based on the degree to which they, in the appropriate order and with or without coaching, perform the actions (Table 18.2).

Evaluative Criteria for Communication With an Elderly Client:
Students will be given feedback based on the degree to which they, in the appropriate order and with or without coaching, perform the actions outlined above (Table 18.3).

18.3 Evaluative Criteria for Communicating With the Elderly Client			
Student Speaking/Listening Behavior	Independent	Prompt	Comments
Client sees "nurse" face in appropriate light			
Normal volume			
Time given for client reflection			
Uses open-ended questions			
Sense of caring conveyed			
Recognition that pain interferes with communication			
Gives explanation related to procedures			
Enunciates consonants			
Uses low-pitched voice			
Addresses physical needs			
Recognizes communication timing			

G. Debriefing Guidelines

Estimated session time is 30 minutes for groups. A general discussion ensues related to the basic skills performed in this scenario. The evaluative criteria in Table 18.2 is used as the foundation. Questions related to technique are encouraged. If videotape is available, the scenario can be reviewed. The area is conducive to participation by all (either group in circle or direct one-to-one seating for an individual and facilitator). The discussion leader is the simulation controller or faculty member. A projector, screen, overhead, or computer is used.

Completed surveys related to beliefs about the elderly are reviewed. This can be done in a number of ways: individual presentation, surveys handed in prior to scenario and tabulated as group data, or automated response anonymous clickers used during the actual discussion. Inferences are solicited about beliefs, assumptions, and resulting behaviors. The discussion leader gives examples of how a belief that "older people are hard of hearing" may lead to shouting or the belief that "older people have no interest in sex" may lead to a disregard in assessment questions. The student or group is guided to focus on positive themes and facts of today's elderly. Stories may be shared as appropriate to objectives and time. The criteria detailed in Table 18.3 is reinforced.

Finally, a review of the 12-item Communication in the Elderly quiz (similar to the survey review style used above) is done.

1. Shouting is required when speaking with older adults. (F)
2. Elderly people hear high-pitch tones easily. (F)
3. Background noise will enhance hearing ability. (F)
4. Light will promote communication. (T)
5. Fatigue, pain, and physical discomfort will influence communication. (T)
6. Hearing aids may need to be turned on, adjusted, or have the battery changed if communication is impaired. (T)
7. Standing off to the side in a shadow facilitates communication. (F)
8. The three-item recall screening asks the assessor to "tell the client to remember three items: apple, table, and dime. Then, a distracting activity is done, and 2 to 3 minutes later, the assessor asks the client what the three items were." (T)
9. Active listening involves reflecting on what a patient has said while listening. (T)
10. Consonants such as: *ch, sw,* or *th* are not heard well as one ages. (T)
11. Attitudes and beliefs influence interactions with elders. (T)
12. Asking elderly clients to bring in their medications (prescription and nonprescription) — the "drug bag" — facilitates accurate assessment of medication intake. (T)

The discussion leader facilitates review of the answers. Rationales are discussed, and participants are encouraged to share what they would continue to do and what they would do differently in future interactions with elderly clients.

H. Suggestions/Key Features to Replicate or Improve

Continue to reinforce learning through constructivist methods such as scaffolding. Use of standard nursing behaviors reinforces and develops confidence in student ability. Refer to Table 18.2.

> *Review of standard nursing behaviors when interacting with a client:* Verification of client orders and plan of care, identification of client, introduction of self and explanation of reason there, asepsis as appropriate, preparation and gathering of equipment/supplies needed, maintenance of privacy and HIPAA standards, appropriate ergonomic/body mechanics when assessing or performing care, maintenance of a safe environment (bed position, call bell, and equipment placement), documentation.

I. Recommendations for Further Use

Complexity can increase in this scenario. Students can develop diagnoses and nursing care plans, and peer evaluation can be done related to outcome attainment and use of nursing process.

In senior-level courses, this scenario can be adapted for use with clients who have neurologic conditions or any type of progressive dementia. Clients with psychiatric conditions may also use this scenario with specific adaptations.

J. Discussion of Simulation-Based Pedagogy and How This New Technology Has Contributed to Improved Student Outcomes

Active learning can promote greater understanding of concepts (Nosich, 2008), higher retention of information (Stice, 1987), and the opportunity to apply knowledge gained through action (Florea & Rafeldt, 2005; Florea, Rafeldt, & Youngblood, 2008). Constructivist learning theory supports simulation in both high and low fidelity. While debriefing is critical to facilitate desired outcomes, educators must remember that incorporation of surveys, discussion, and NCLEX-RN–style questions will also contribute to efficient internalization of content and resulting practice as a student nurse and future registered nurse.

References

Florea, M., & Rafeldt, L. (2005). *Information literacy for nurses*. Presentation at North East American Library Association Conference, Boston, MA.

Florea, M., Rafeldt, L., & Youngblood, S. (2008). Using an information literacy program to prepare nursing students to practice in a virtual workplace. In: P. Zemliansky & K. St. Amant (Eds.), *Handbook of research on virtual workplaces and the new nature of business practices* (pp. 317–333) Hershey, PA: IGA Global.

National Council of State Boards of Nursing. (2007). *NCLEX-RN examination: Test plan for the national council licensure examination for registered nurses*. Retrieved June 18, 2008, from https://www.ncsbn.org/RN_Test_Plan_2007_Web.pdf

Nosich, G. (2008). *Learning to think things through: A guide to critical thinking across the curriculum* (3rd ed.). Upper Saddle River, NJ: Prentice Hall.

Stice, J. (1987). Using Kolb's learning cycle to improve student learning. *Engineering Education, 77*(5), 291–296.

Vygotsky, L.S. (1978). *Thought and language*. Cambridge: Massachusetts Institute of Technology.

Recommended Readings

Ackley, B., & Ladwig, G. (2008). *Nursing diagnosis handbook: An evidence-based guide to planning care* (8th ed.). St. Louis, MO: Mosby.

Benner, P. (2001). *From novice to expert: Excellence and power in clinical nursing practice*. Upper Saddle River, NJ: Prentice Hall.

Dillon, P. (2007). *Nursing health assessment: A critical thinking case studies approach* (2nd ed.). Philadelphia, PA: F.A. Davis Company.

Ebersole, P., Hess, P., Touhy, T., Jett, K., & Luggen, A. (2008). *Toward healthy aging: Human needs and nursing response* (7th ed.). St. Louis, MO: Mosby.

Fessey, V. (2007). Patients who present with dementia: Exploring the knowledge of hospital nurses. *Nursing Older People, 19*(10), 29–33.

Giordano, J., & Deckinger, E. (2003). Guidelines for communicating with our most elderly. *Academic Exchange Quarterly.* Retrieved January 17, 2008, from http://www.rapidintellect.com/AEQweb/mo2401fe04.htm

Hogan, M. (2008). Therapeutic communication and environment. In M. Hogan (Ed.), *Comprehensive review for NCLEX-RN: Reviews and rationales* (pp. 269–283). Upper Saddle River, NJ: Prentice Hall.

Jeffries, P. (2007). *Simulation in nursing education: From conceptualization to evaluation.* New York: National League for Nursing.

Rafeldt, L. (2008). Age-related care of older adults. In M. Hogan (Ed.), *Comprehensive review for NCLEX-RN: Reviews and rationales* (pp. 254–268). Upper Saddle River, NJ: Prentice Hall.

Smeltzer, S., Bare, B., Hinkle, J., & Cheever, K. (2008). *Brunner & Suddarth's textbook of medical-surgical nursing* (11th ed.). Philadelphia: Lippincott Williams & Wilkins.

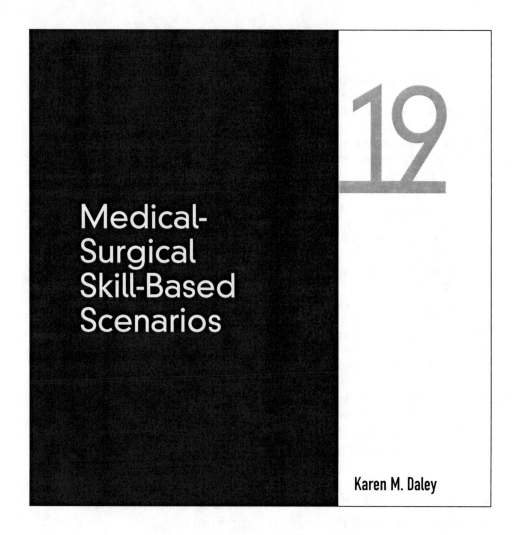

Medical-Surgical Skill-Based Scenarios

19

Karen M. Daley

A. Discussion of Implementation of Simulation-Based Pedagogy in Each Contributor's Individualized Teaching

At Western Connecticut State University, nursing students complete three levels of medical-surgical courses, each with increasing breadth and complexity. The first course introduces common medical diagnoses found in chronic illness, long-term care, and restorative subacute care. In the middle medical surgical course, students are introduced to common diagnoses requiring surgical intervention. In the third course, nursing care and interventions for complex patients such as intensive care patients are studied within the context of the nursing process. Although the theory has been introduced in the foundation course, the second course is the first to include task and skill training related to acute care. Traditionally performed on static task trainers, current nursing students have begun using a multipronged approach to task training. In the seminar portion of this middle surgical course, students are given the opportunity to read and review these skills in text and video. Instructors then demonstrate these skills in seminar and allow students to practice on static task trainers and manikins. In evaluations of the courses in the past, students did not seem to make the theory-seminar-clinical connections needed to transfer this knowledge as an integrated whole to their nursing practice. With a multipronged approach of read/study, view, and practice, however, we have found that the imbedding of skills within a scenario or a case study that has been transformed into a scenario for use with a human patient simulator (HPS) was beneficial and increased their confidence in performing the skill on actual patients.

In addressing this need within a traditional nursing laboratory, an eight-bed nursing lab without computer or Internet access was renovated into a computer projection and instructor station with four student-use computers with Internet access and four beds with manikins. Videos of skills available online could then be projected and discussed by instructors and teachers, then reaccessed by students during open lab practice. In addition, these skill videos are available for students to view from home computers.

With the purchase of the Department of Nursing's first HPS, a section of the lab was designated as the simulation area, and over time, equipment was purchased to enhance the "realness" and usability of the area for simulation. A bed was taken out and replaced by a stretcher to make the HPS more mobile. Several small grants and summer curriculum funds provided both the equipment organization and time for constructing skill-based scenarios to match the existing skill-training modules. In addition, several more grants allowed updates and upgrades to the HPS as the technology became available. Although not utilized consistently by all faculty teaching the course, the availability of this high-fidelity learning tool gives each instructor the flexibility to teach at different levels of technology to meet student needs.

B. Description of Educational Materials Available in Your Teaching Area and Relative to Your Specialty

As described previously, the simulation area used for these simulations is embedded in an existing nursing lab. It is an open area, with the HPS residing on a stretcher with an IV machine and pole nearby. Also in this area is a treatment cart that has become the simulation cart. In this cart are all the supplies needed for mock-up of the scenarios and exclusively for use with the HPS. There are three hospital beds with static manikins and multiple partial task trainer manikins available, such as a pelvic model for urinary catheter insertion. Weekly objectives for the modules direct students and instructors to the equipment needed for each scheduled seminar. Each seminar coincides with a nursing concept being taught in the theory portion of the course. For example, when teaching about pain and comfort concepts in theory/class, students are asked in seminar to review pain assessments, interventions to enhance a patient's comfort level, and evaluative criteria by which to judge the success of nursing interventions for the surgical patient. Taught as individual tasks, students learn how to administer shots and give IV pain medications. On the HPS within a scenario, students can interact with the HPS, assess the pain level of the "patient," decide which medication is appropriate, and measure the effectiveness of the medication. Unlike the static task training, the use of the HPS allows for practice with therapeutic communication and may involve contacting other health care professionals and possibly dealing with a patient with varying levels of pain relief. Safety techniques can be overlaid as well by asking the student to check the five rights, put up side rails for the sedated patient, and concurrently assess the effects of the narcotic medications on the patient's respiratory system.

Five scenarios were created to supplement and complement learning within the seminar portion of the medical-surgical course (Nursing 255). This chapter presents these scenarios. Scenarios have similar objectives and expected outcomes based on the nursing process. Initially written as computerized scenarios with computer programming, each was rewritten with additional summer curriculum funds to better reflect the need of instructors and students for flexibility in implementing the scenarios. Currently, these scenarios are written as "on the fly" with the instructor running the scenario. Each scenario is simple and task oriented and is written to bring to life the common surgical nursing interventions.

At Western Connecticut State University, we do not have lab personnel, so each simulation must be run by an instructor who is trained in simulation. In some instances, this has resulted in the instructor enthusiastically jumping in with both feet to learn and utilize simulation. For others, lack of time and training opportunities are most often cited for nonuse of simulation. In addition, the classic task-training method is still a tried-and-true method of effective teaching for most students, although students are requesting more simulation in this course each year.

C. Specific Objective for Simulation Utilization Within a Specific Course and the Overall Program

1. Student will use the nursing process to assess and intervene in a common surgical nursing problem.
2. Student will develop a basic level competency in performing a surgical nursing intervention.

D. Introduction of Scenario to Include Setting the Scene, Technology Used, Objectives, and Description of Participants

Setting the Scene

Each scenario includes a list of necessary equipment and supplies to mock up the HPS. These supplies are available in the simulation cart.

Technology Used

High-fidelity HPS

Objectives

1. Student will use the nursing process to identify a surgical nursing problem that needs intervention.
2. Student will practice a selected skill within a scenario that integrates maintaining a standard of care, therapeutic communication, safety precautions, and psychosocial care.

The Association of Colleges of Nursing *Essentials of Baccalaureate Education for Professional Nursing Practice* (AACN, 2007) item addressed in the simulation includes the following:

Essential IX: Baccalaureate Generalist Nursing Practice

The National Council of State Boards of Nursing's National Council Licensure Examination for Registered Nurses (NCLEX-RN) test plan categories and subcategories (NCSBN, 2007) addressed in the simulation include the following:

Safe and Effective Care Environment
> *Management of Care*
>> Delegation
>> Establishing Priorities
>> Ethical Practice
>> Informed Consent
>> Legal Rights and Responsibilities
> *Safety and Infection Control*
>> Medical and Surgical Asepsis
>> Standard/Transmission-Based/Other Precautions
>> Safe Use of Equipment

Health Promotion and Maintenance
>> Techniques of Physical Assessment

Psychosocial Integrity
>> Coping Mechanisms
>> Therapeutic Communications
>> Unexpected Body Image Changes

Physiological Integrity
> *Basic Care and Comfort*
>> Elimination
>> Non-Pharmacological Comfort Interventions
>> Personal Hygiene
>> Rest and Sleep
> *Pharmacological and Parenteral Therapies*
>> Dosage Calculation
>> Expected Effects/Outcomes
>> Medication Administration
>> Parenteral/Intravenous Therapies
>> Pharmacological Agents/Actions
>> Pharmacological Pain Management

Reduction of Risk Potential
    Diagnostic Tests
    Laboratory Values
    Potential for Complications of Diagnostic Tests/Treatments/
        Procedures
    System Specific Assessments
    Therapeutic Procedures
    Vital Signs
Physiological Adaptation
    Hemodynamics
    Illness Management

Participants: In these simple scenarios, the only participants are a small group of three to four nursing students and the HPS. Students seem to prefer this in contrast to be being "put on the spot" one by one. Students can portray: a team of nurses using group process to decide on care of the patients, or staff, or family members played by additional nursing students or faculty.

E. Describe Running of the Scenario

Each seminar topic area runs either 1 or 2 weeks for 3 hours each. The first hour usually involves discussion and application of the surgical concept being taught in class. The discussion involves taking that concept through the nursing process by integrating previously learned concepts with the new and reviewing common nursing interventions needed for the surgical patient in that topic area. During the second hour, the associated tasks are demonstrated, and the remaining time is given to the students for supervised practice. Students arrive ready to practice, having reviewed the skill content, viewed the associated videos, and, in the best case, having already tried to practice at home with their nursing kit.

    During the designated practice time, two instructors are available to help with skills. When one is trained in the use of the HPS, that instructor works with the students who are ready to embed the skill into a scenario. The HPS is set up prior to the beginning of the scenario, and the scenario begins just as if you were going to walk into a room to care for a patient. Students should identify and introduce themselves, check the identity of the patient, and begin a surgical assessment. During the assessment, a common surgical problem is found and will need interventions to address the problem. A skill will have to be performed to alleviate the problem and evaluation of the intervention will follow.

F. Presentation of Completed Template

The following five medical-surgical skill-based scenarios have been included based on those written for this course. The scenario template is somewhat different from the templates used throughout the book in order to show the original "as written" format that is currently in use at the University.

NUR 255—Scenario #1
Surgical Pain (Skill: Administration of Pain Medications)

Title: Surgical Pain

63-year-old man admitted yesterday for a left knee replacement. He is 1 day postop. During the student's morning assessment, he complains of pain.

Equipment Needed:

> IV setup
> Syringe for pain meds
> Stethoscope
> Ace wrap for left knee

Objectives:

1. Student will be able to identify source and level of pain.
2. Student will perform appropriate assessments in order to accurately assess pain level.
3. Student will correctly intervene to treat pain.

Settings for Patient:

> HR: 108
> SpO$_2$: 93
> CO$_2$: 34
> Temp: 37.2°C
> RR: 20
> BP: 96/64
> Vocals: "I've never had pain like this before!"

Interventions:

_____ Identify self and patient.
_____ Identify purpose of visit.
_____ Perform surgical assessment.
_____ Check incision.
_____ Check vital signs.
_____ Change BP to 110/80
_____ Vocals: "I don't feel well!"
_____ Assess pain on pain scale.
_____ Check Dr. orders; select and administer IV pain meds.
_____ Evaluate effectiveness.
_____ Reposition patient with safety precautions for sedation.

Settings:

> HR: 80
> SpO$_2$: 98
> RR: 12
> BP: 120/80
> Vocals: I feel better now." Repeat × 1.

Evaluation:
Patient states, "I feel better now." Level of pain <5.

NUR 255—Scenario #2

Hypovolemia (Skill: Administration of Parenteral Fluids)

Title: Hypovolemia
55 year-old woman, 2 days postop abdominal surgery with large open wound. Wound is draining large amounts of serosanguinous fluid, patient is NPO with a nasogastric (NG) tube.

Equipment Needed:

IV setup
Stethoscope
Red, soaked abdominal wound dressing with drainage
NG tube

Objectives:

1. Student will recognize need for overall assessment of patient and then recognize the signs and symptoms of hypovolemia.
2. Student will choose correct IV fluid and recognize need to hydrate patient.
3. Student will evaluate interventions appropriately.

Settings for the Patient:

HR: 80
SpO$_2$: 98
T: 37.2°C
BP: 100/80

Interventions:

_____ Identify self and patient.
_____ Identify purpose of visit.
_____ Perform surgical assessment.
_____ Check IV.
_____ O$_2$ in place.
_____ Cardiac monitor on.
_____ Check tubes/wound.
_____ Increase HR to 92.
_____ Change BP to 90/72.
_____ Vocals: "I feel dizzy."
_____ Reposition patient to low Fowler.
_____ Check VS, assess wound, check labs, check I & O.
_____ Vocals: "I don't feel well."
_____ Redress wound, and assess IV fluid rate and solution. Choose appropriate solution and rate.
_____ Check orders for antibiotic/anti-infective. Administer as ordered.
_____ Change BP to 120/80, RR to 12, HR to 80.

_____ Document findings.
_____ Vocals: "I feel better now."

Evaluation:
Patient reports feeling better, and BP returns to normal

NUR 255—Scenario #3

Wound Assessment (Skill: Surgical Wound Dressing Change)

Title: Wound Assessment
57-year-old man, 1 day postop with open cholecystectomy. Patient has large abdominal dressing with Montgomery straps and a Hemovac drain.

Equipment Needed:

Montgomery straps with dressing
Hemovac drain
Stethoscope

Objectives:

1. Student will assess wound for signs and symptoms of healing or infection.
2. Student will perform appropriate interventions.
3. Student will evaluate wound and effectiveness of interventions.

Settings for Patient:

HR: 80
SpO$_2$: 98
T: 37.2°C
RR: 10
BP: 120/80

Interventions:

_____ Identify self and patient.
_____ Identify purpose of visit.
_____ Perform surgical assessment.
_____ Check that IV is running, oxygen and monitor are on.
_____ Check tubes.
_____ Edema check.
_____ Check pulse.
_____ Check dressing.
_____ Assess wound.
_____ Vocals: Moaning
_____ Redress wound, check labs, check I & O.
_____ Administer anti-infective, document findings.
_____ Vocals: "Thank you."

Evaluation:

Student accurately assesses healing of surgical wound.
Student redresses wound with surgical asepsis.

NUR 255—Scenario #4

Hypoxia (Skill: Administration of Supplemental Oxygen)

Title: Hypoxia

60-year-old woman, 1 day postop with right mastectomy. Patient has a large Ace wrap bandage around upper rib cage and a Jackson Pratt drain. Patient is receiving IV morphine for pain.

Equipment Needed:

>   Stethoscope
>   Pulse oximeter
> O_2 setup
>   JP drain
>   IV setup

Objectives:

1. Student will assess for and recognize signs and symptoms of hypoxia.
2. Student will intervene to treat hypoxia.
3. Student will evaluate interventions appropriately.

Settings for Patient:

>   Bilateral wheezes at volume 9
> SpO_2: 88
>   RR: 22
>   BP: 140/86
>   Vocals: Cough, repeat × 1

Interventions:

_____ Identify self and patient.
_____ Identify purpose of visit.
_____ Perform surgical assessment.
_____ Focused respiratory assessment and auscultate lungs.
_____ Vocals: "I don't feel well."
_____ Reposition patient with head of bed elevated.
_____ Obtain pulse oximetry.
_____ Administer oxygen: Select oxygen delivery device per standard of care.
_____ Review technique with patient the "Cough and Deep Breathe." Have patient demonstrate and perform per protocol.
_____ Review and have patient perform incentive spirometry per protocol.
_____ Obtain pulse oximetry.
_____ Re-evaluate patient with focused respiratory assessment.
_____ Change wheezes bilateral to volume 5, and increase SpO_2 to 99.
_____ Vocals: "I feel better now."

Evaluation:

Student able to assess and treat hypoxia without progressing.

NUR 255—Scenario #5

Urinary Retention (Skill: Urinary Catheterization)

Title: Urinary Retention

63-year-old man, 1 day postop right knee replacement. Patient has a large Ace wrap bandage around right knee with a compression dressing in place. Patient was receiving IV morphine for pain on a PCA that was discontinued this morning. He has now been on pain pills for 8 hours and has not been able to void since catheter was removed 6 hours ago.

Equipment Needed:

> IV setup with PCA
> Urinary catheter kit
> Urinal
> Ultrasound probe to do a bladder scan

Objectives:

1. Student will assess for and recognize signs and symptoms of urinary retention.
2. Student will intervene to perform bladder scan and urinary catheterization.
3. Student will evaluate interventions appropriately.

Settings for Patient:

> SpO$_2$: 98
> RR: 16
> BP: 140/86
> HR: 72

Interventions:

_____ Identify self and patient.
_____ Identify purpose of visit.
_____ Perform surgical assessment.
_____ Vocals: "I feel full, but I cannot seem to use the urinal."
_____ Assess bladder with bladder scan. Results: 650 cc urine in the bladder.
_____ Explain reason for urinary catheterization and reposition patient.
_____ Perform urinary catheterization.
_____ Assess color and quantity of urine. Document.
_____ Vocals: "I feel better now."

Evaluation:
Student able to assess and treat urinary retention

G. Debriefing Guidelines

Instructors may want to consider these reflection questions for use routinely after the implementation of the skill-based scenarios:

1. Was the correct nursing problem identified and addressed?
2. Were medical and, if needed, surgical asepsis maintained? How?
3. Did the nurse communicate effectively with the patients about the nursing problem and the interventions needed?
4. Were safety precautions taken at all times?
5. Did the implementation of the skill follow the standard of care described in the skill book?
6. In reflecting on the implementation of this scenario with real patients, what additional postsurgical problems would contribute to the assessment and implementation of your nursing intervention? In addition, what psychosocial issues may also need to be addressed in the postsurgical patient?
7. What was done well? What could be improved?

H. Suggestions/Key Features to Replicate or Improve

As stated previously, these scenarios have not been fully implemented in this course due to time and training. Each year, more instructors try some of the scenarios. In addition, an instructor that specializes in HPS technology offers to work with the students during open lab time as requested by students. The HPS has also been used after or as part of clinical time, which allows for a more focused interaction with students as a group. Use of these scenarios is a work in progress, as is true of many scenario implementations. Each year, more is added to improve the scenarios. The debriefing questions added above will be used for the first time as written this year.

I. Recommendations for Further Use

Keeping the scenario as simple as possible is important at this point in the student's education. Skill competency is essential as these students move forward. At the end of the semester, the students must pass a skill practicum in order to pass the course. The HPS has been available for use as an option for skill testing in this skill practicum. Using the HPS on a more routine basis with these skills may provide the opportunity for students to learn skills in context by integrating patient interaction, therapeutic communication, safety precautions, and use of the nursing process within a scenario. In addition, frequent exposure to the HPS throughout this semester increases the student's comfort level in interacting with the simulator as a learning tool.

J. Discussion of Simulation-Based Pedagogy and How This New Technology Has Contributed to Improved Student Outcomes

Students report that they enjoy interacting with the HPS and practicing "real" surgical patient situations prior to seeing these problems arise in clinical. Instructors in these seminars emphasize that these skill-based seminars are a safe place to learn and ask questions so that students enthusiastically try and re-try to achieve the standard of care for each of the skills required. Within the context of a scenario, instructors are able to view student implementation of the nursing process step by step. In clinical, students often seek out instructors only after an assessment has been made that a surgical nursing problem needs to be addressed. From these perspectives, simulation-based skill/task training has improved student outcomes by increasing student confidence in their ability to perform selected nursing skills and increased instructor confidence in the student ability to accurately implement the nursing process in relation to selected surgical nursing skills. Embedding the skills in a scenario enables the student to enact the role of the nurse not only from a task-oriented view but also taking into consideration holistic patient care.

References

American Association of Colleges of Nursing. (2007). The October 22, 2007 draft of the *essentials of baccalaureate education for professional nursing practice.* Washington, DC: Author.

National Council of State Boards of Nursing. (2007). *NCLEX-RN examination: Test plan for the national council licensure examination for registered nurses.* Retrieved June 18, 2007, from https://www.ncsbn.org/RN_Test_Plan_2007_Web.pdf

Recommended Texts

Deglin, J., & Vallerand, A. (2007). *Davis's drug guide for nurses* (11th ed.). Philadelphia: F.A. Davis.

Doenges, M., Moorehouse, P., & Murr, D. (2006). *Nursing care plans: Guidelines for individualizing client care across the life span* (7th ed.). St. Louis: F.A. Davis.

Fischbach, F. (2008). *A manual of laboratory and diagnostic tests* (9th ed.). Philadelphia: Lippincott.

Perry, P. (2005). *Clinical nursing skills and techniques* (6th ed.). St. Louis, MO: Mosby.

Potter, P., & Perry, A.G. (2005). *Fundamentals of nursing* (6th ed.). St. Louis, MO: Mosby.

Smeltzer, S. C., & Bare, B. (2008). *Textbook of medical-surgical nursing* (11th ed.). New York: Lippincott Williams & Wilkins.

20

Undergraduate Senior Capstone Scenarios: Pearls, Pitfalls, and Politics

Laura T. Gantt and
Robin Webb Corbett

This chapter will address the development of a scenario and the use of scenarios in a senior capstone course. Faculty and student responsibilities will be reviewed. Documentation of patient assessment and nursing interventions are included in the scenario.

Nursing simulation is relatively new, but its growth has been exponential. Faculty commonly use low-fidelity simulators to teach nursing care. Many faculty are interested in the use of high-fidelity simulators, but information is lacking regarding simulation scenarios and pertinent "how-to's."

A. Discussion of Implementation of Simulation-Based Pedagogy in Each Contributor's Individualized Teaching

The clinical capstone coordinator had been on the forefront of online courses that couple audio with slides and animations of complex subjects, such as the hypothalamic-pituitary-ovarian axis. While faculty lacked the technologic expertise, they previously had the opportunity to work with an information technologist who was also curious and willing to experiment and learn during the process. The marriage of content expertise and technologic expertise resulted in two online physiology courses.

B. Description of Educational Materials Available in Your Teaching Area and Relative to Your Specialty

In the summer of 2006, East Carolina University College of Nursing (CON) relocated to the new Health Sciences Complex. The new building has eight simulation laboratories with a new executive director of Learning Technologies and Labs. Previously, the Concepts Integration Lab (CIL) had been one room with one adult high-fidelity human patient simulator (HPS), one child medium-fidelity HPS, and one birthing simulator. These simulators had been used minimally. In contrast, now with expanded space and human and other resources, the CON purchased several infant, child, and adult HPS in addition to a variety of static manikins.

C. Specific Objective for Simulation Utilization Within a Specific Course and the Overall Program

Prior to the beginning of the school year, the clinical capstone coordinator met with lab personnel to plan critical-thinking scenarios. How naive we were! Yes, we knew it would be time intensive, but little did we know about the nuts and bolts of scenario development and implementation or how much faculty consternation would result. But we proceeded.

In meeting with the senior clinical capstone faculty, numerous issues were voiced. These issues included concerns about evaluation, scheduling, student readiness, staffing, scenario planning, and skill templates. In addition, nursing administration voiced concerns regarding the complexity of the scenarios, believing the scenarios needed to be more in line with a patient cardiac arrest or mock code. Finally, however, support from the Dean of CON allowed us the opportunity to implement the scenarios. As part of the process, the executive director of the labs and the course coordinator developed a research component as part of the student evaluations.

Previously in the clinical capstone course, only 120 clinical hours were required in addition to a 2-hour seminar. One hour of the seminar was for faculty demonstration of clinical nursing skills and techniques review, and 1 hour was for dialogue regarding their precepted clinical experiences. Quizzes were done each week following the nursing skills presentation to facilitate learning. At that time, students had access to IV equipment, tubes, drains, blood transfusion equipment and supplies, high- and low-fidelity HPS, and static manikins but generally only went to lab to practice when mandated by the faculty in response to a faculty–preceptor meeting or preceptor concern. Students voiced concerns that there were limited opportunities to perform nursing skills, such as insertion of a nasogastric (NG) tube, during clinical rotations. In addition, due to increasing enrollment in our program as well as surrounding nursing programs, clinical sites had become overloaded; lab sections also had increased numbers of students.

The coordinators for the final-semester senior nursing courses were concerned regarding nursing agency comments specific to the problems that graduates of the program demonstrated related to critical thinking, time management, organizational abilities, and performance of nursing skills or tasks. These faculty purported that simulation scenarios would enable students to practice skills and reinforce critical thinking. In contrast to being "just a skills review," the simulation would engage the student learner.

For the clinical capstone faculty, engagement theory undergirds the process of learning in the scenarios (Haworth & Conrad, 1997). Components of engagement theory as discussed by Haworth & Conrad (1977) include the concepts of relate, create, and donation. Students *relate* via their collaboration in the development of decision-making and clinical skills. As a course assignment, students relate to each other and faculty as they learn the relationships among critical thinking, establishing priorities, and decision making in the patient care scenarios. Students must identify important aspects of patient care and select the most appropriate manner in which to complete their scenario. These collaborative endeavors include review of the principles prior to the scenarios with competency check sheets, discussion of clinical priorities and critical thinking in precepted clinical experiences, and weekly seminars. Students *create* through developing learning contracts specific to their learning needs. For example, students frequently identify critical thinking, clinical skills, establishing clinical priorities, and documentation as learning needs prior to their precepted clinicals. In addition, students, faculty, and staff nurses collaboratively identify clinical skills for the scenarios.

Thus, the six clinical nursing skills and techniques for the clinical capstone course include starting an IV fluid, administering IV push or piggyback medication, administering a blood transfusion, insertion of NG tube and administering NG medication, tracheostomy care and suctioning, maintaining sterile procedure, and demonstrating isolation procedure. With each scenario, as the student performs the clinical nursing skill, a common problem occurs (i.e., the oxygen saturation rate drops to below 90 mm Hg, and the pulse rate goes up as the student suctions a tracheostomy), mandating critical thinking and problem solving by the student. *Donation* refers to the critical review by their faculty and their self-review in their scenario debriefing. The evaluation debriefing begins with the faculty asking, "What do you think you did well?" This question is then followed by "What would you like to do differently?"

In addition, students document in a narrative format the clinical scenario with the instructions to document "as in clinical." Students are then asked to evaluate the clinical activity via an objective tool (Chambers, 2006) followed by a subjective measure of "What was most helpful to you in this experience? What could have been done to facilitate learning in this experience?" Specifically, students include in the clinical scenario evaluation those scenario characteristics that contributed to their learning of critical thinking, decision making, and clinical skills as well as recommendations for future scenarios. Therefore, they relate past learning clinical activities to their clinical scenarios.

Initially, the Capstone Critical Thinking Simulation Comprehensive Scenarios were planned *not* to focus on nursing skills. Faculty "assumed" that senior students came with this knowledge. However, numerous faculty were teaching nursing fundamentals, and there was a lack of a guiding clinical nursing skills and techniques checklist. It was noted that many students had learned different techniques in performing nursing skills. Cognizant that different techniques are correct, students requested that faculty provide them with "one way" to perform a certain skill, such as insertion of an NG tube. Therefore, the clinical capstone coordinator, in collaboration with the lab's personnel and the nursing fundamentals faculty coordinators, reviewed numerous clinical nursing skills and techniques. While pertinent, none were found to be succinct and concise. In previous teaching endeavors, the clinical capstone coordinator had worked with another School of Nursing colleague who had an effective and dynamic nursing simulation program. When contacted, the nursing colleague willingly shared her agency's competency checklist and materials with permission to modify them as needed. The competency checklists were adapted after review by the nursing fundamentals and medical-surgical faculty, as well as CON nursing administrators. Competency checklist notebooks were placed in the Learning Resource Center (LRC) and in each lab. In addition, competency checklists were placed on the clinical capstone Blackboard, the online course medium for our university.

Information shared with the students prior to the scenario is listed below:

The Clinical Capstone Critical Thinking Simulation Comprehensive Scenario will assess your ability to perform selected nursing skills appropriately in clinical scenarios. Evaluation of the clinical scenarios will include skill performance, critical thinking, time management, organization of care, documentation, and patient/staff safety. This will be a 30-minute scenario, and the time will be from your clinical hours (Note: 126 clinical hours).

Reference materials are available in the LRC and via your textbooks and *** materials. These materials include the key concepts and procedures of the skills with specific information related to skills. These materials will be located in the LRC and the skills lab in a notebook for your review. The *** Nursing Skills CD-ROM is located on the LRC computers. In addition, you have the *** PLAN A Basic Nursing Skills DVD.

The appointment schedule for the scenarios will be posted. Skills will include those listed below and may include other skills. More information will be shared at your scheduled seminar.

Skills:
Oxygen administration and care
Blood administration and care
Chest tube insertion and care
Intravenous therapy, to include starting an IV, hanging an IV piggyback, troubleshooting, IV medication administration, and care after medication administration
NG tube insertion, tube feedings, medication administration, and care
Tracheostomy care and suctioning
Care of the patient in isolation
Foley catheter insertion and care

Practice Times:
You are encouraged to practice these skills in the CILs prior to your assigned check off.
     You may make an appointment to practice these skills with CIL personnel at ***-****-**** or e-mail Mrs. *** at ***. You will need to contact the CIL at least 24 to 48 hours prior to the time you wish to schedule an appointment.

Simulation Scenarios:
Thirty-minute appointments will be made for you based on the posted schedule and your schedule.
     Re-Evaluation times will be scheduled for students as needed.

As many students had never worked with a high-fidelity simulator before, simulation lab orientation sessions were planned in larger groups of 10 to 20 students. Thirty-minute orientation periods allowed students to acquaint themselves with the abilities of the simulator; they could see and hear it and have their questions answered. Handouts were distributed that listed attributes of the simulator and labs. Equipment and supplies were placed in carts and mobile units to "simulate" a nursing unit for the scenarios and open lab practice sessions.

Course objectives for the senior clinical capstone course are as follows:

1. Demonstrate competency as a beginning professional nurse in the following roles:
   - Care provider
   - Collaborator
   - Coordinator
   - Manager
   - Educator
   - Consumer of research
2. Use effective leadership skills, including the following:
   - Priority setting
   - Delegation
   - Conflict management
   - Decision making
   - Communication
3. Incorporate appropriate theoretical concepts and research findings that enhance high-quality, evidence-based professional nursing care to clients.
4. Implement interventions that foster client, interdisciplinary team, and organizational goals and objectives.

Capstone clinical faculty believed that all objectives supported the use of simulation in this course. For all scenarios, the American Association of Colleges of Nursing *Essentials of Baccalaureate Education for Professional Nursing Practice* (AACN, 2007) items addressed includes the following:

Essential IX: Baccalaureate Generalist Nursing Practice

For all scenarios, the National Council of State Boards of Nursing's National Council Licensure Examination for Registered Nurses (NCSBN-RN) test plan categories and subcategories (NCSBN, 2007) addressed include the following:

Safe, Effective Care Environment
    Management of Care
        Establishing Priorities
    Safety and Infection Control
        Standard/Transmission-Based/Other Precautions
        Error Prevention
Physiological Integrity
    Pharmacological and Parenteral Therapies
        Adverse Effects/Contraindications
        Expected Effects/Outcomes
        Medication Administration
        Pharmacological Pain Management
        Dosage Calculation
        Parenteral/Intravenous Therapies
    Reduction of Risk Potential
        Laboratory Values
        Vital Signs
        System Specific Assessment
    Physiological Adaptation
        Unexpected Response to Therapies

D. Introduction of Scenario to Include Setting the Scene, Technology Used, Objectives, and Description of Participants

The following scenario template can be used as a practice scenario or an evaluative scenario.

Title: Clinical Capstone Critical Thinking Simulation Comprehensive Scenario

Focus Area: Medical-surgical Graduating Senior Scenario

These scenarios are part of the last-semester capstone course for traditional undergraduate BSN students. Students actually complete *one of six* medical-surgical scenarios.

Scenario Description:
The patient is a 76-year-old retired white female of average height and weight admitted to the hospital with acute onset of nausea and vomiting. Patient history includes right medullary cerebrovascular accident with mild residual left-sided weakness, diabetes mellitus, hypertension, dysphagia, status post percutaneous endoscopic gastrostomy placement, urinary tract infection, and anemia. The patient has no allergies, and home medications include currently Aggrenox, Amoxicillin, Pronestyl, Aldomet, and NPH insulin. Her mental status is within normal limits, and she has been living with her daughter in Goldsboro in a

one-story home with three steps to enter and handrails. She denies any alcohol or tobacco use.

Each of the six possible scenarios is based on the same patient history with the "patient" having developed a series of problems and complications as she moves through the hospital system. The nursing student assumes the role of the RN receiving report on one of her patients. A nursing report was generated for each scenario and orally given by the faculty following the students' "random draw" for their scenario. Students were given instructions that their scenario would last no longer than 20 minutes, with 10 minutes for debriefing; students were asked if they would like to be notified when they had 5 minutes left in their allotted scenario time. Students could request assistance or needed supplies from a staff nurse or unlicensed assistive personnel (UAP) via the bed "call" button. Play phones were available for students to contact the physician or physician extender, with the faculty answering and playing the role of the physician or physician extender.

E & F. Describe Running of the Scenario and Presentation of Completed Template

As mentioned previously, students performed one of six scenarios below:

Scenario 1: On initial patient admission, the nurse receives report from the nurse going off shift. The nurse reporting off states that the patient assessment is normal except for mild abdominal distention and hypoactive bowel sounds. Laboratory tests to include complete blood count and chemistry panel are reported to have been drawn with results pending. The patient's health care provider has written orders for the patient to be scheduled for a CT scan. There are also orders for the patient to have an IV inserted and receive IV promethazine (Phenergan) for nausea.

Scenario 2: The "patient" experiences ongoing nausea and vomiting and is made NPO. The nurse receives orders to increase the IV fluids, call a GI physician consult, place an NG tube and connect it to low wall suction, and give a pain med via NG tube for pain.

Scenario 3: After the consultation with the GI physician, the "patient" is diagnosed with a GI bleed. The patient's hematocrit and hemoglobin indicate bleeding, and the patient has orders for a transfusion, additional lab work after the transfusion, and IV pain medication. The patient has a transfusion reaction.

Scenario 4: After the "patient" has the transfusion reaction, she continues to deteriorate and is eventually intubated. In this scenario, she has had a tracheostomy and needs suctioning. She also has orders for IV antibiotics for pneumonia.

Scenario 5: The "patient" has increased abdominal pain. The physician writes orders to replace the patient's NG tube. There are also orders for IV pain meds.

Scenario 6: The "patient" has developed a fever and is thought to have a UTI and an infection (MRSA or VRE) requiring isolation. There are orders for urinalysis with culture and isolation.

The following is an example of the report given to the nursing student before the beginning of scenario 2:

Ms. Edna Echo, a 76 yo WF, in room 301, was admitted this am at 0500 for evaluation of ongoing nausea and vomiting. She is a patient of Dr. King, who is requesting a GI consult by Dr. Stein. They suspect a GI bleed.

Ms. Echo is now NPO due to increased vomiting during the day. She remains on bed rest.

She had a CBC and Chem 7 drawn at 0600. Some results are pending.

Ms. Echo has a CT of the abdomen scheduled for today.

IV fluids in right antecubital—NS @ 75cc/h.

Pain is 8 on scale of 1–10; "abdominal" and "sharp."

Nausea now 3 on scale of 1−10.

Vomited approx 300 cc reddish-brown emesis and is guaiac positive.

Labs: Anemia, Hct = 24—related to questionable GI bleed.

Assessment: Normal, excluding abdomen more distended and more tender than 0900 assessment.

Orders to Be Done:
NPO.
Increase IV NS to 125 cc/h.
Insert NG and place to LWS.
Administer Percocet 1 tab × 1 per NG for abdominal pain.
Guaiac all stools.
Contact Dr. Stein for GI consult.

Setting the Scene:

Equipment needed:

■ High-fidelity HPS with patient gown; identification band; gender-appropriate body parts; and optional wig, glasses, and other props.
■ Audio-video recording device
■ Medical equipment (patient monitor, pulse oximeter, blood pressure cuff, oxygen hookup and flow meter, suction with canister and tubing for low wall suction, stethoscope)
■ Sink for hand washing and/or waterless hand cleaner
■ Medical supply cart with supplies and/or practice medications (stethoscope, NG tubes, Toomey syringes, medicine cups, tape, pH paper, suction, IV supplies, practice Percocet, medicine crusher, sterile water, watch or clock
■ Medical record (patient chart to include orders, progress notes, laboratory values)

Resources needed:
Drug resource book, paper and pen for performing drug and IV calculations, textbooks, nursing report scripts

Participant roles:
1 student, 1 faculty to observe and evaluate, 1 simulator operator (staff, faculty, or instructional technology personnel); other roles such as staff nurse, physician or physician extender, and unlicensed assistive personnel may be added.

Initial Settings for the Human Patient Simulator
See Table 20.1 for initial settings related to six capstone scenarios.

Required Student Assessments and Actions
Focused patient assessment, communication, skills accomplishment according to the competency checklist, medication administration if appropriate to scenario, problem solving related to changes in patient status, reassessment as necessary

Instructor Interventions
The instructor may ask the students if they would like to call for nursing assistance using the "call" bell if they appear to need assistance, if they would like the UAP to bring them supplies or equipment using the "call" bell, or if they would like to contact the physician or physician extender via the "play" phone.

Evaluative Criteria:
Initially, the students were evaluated on the scenario using the competency checklists described and a grading system to accompany the checklists. The grading system was at 5-point intervals dependent on the number of errors. Interrater reliability was developed with faculty reviewing the competency checklists to determine critical items for scoring. Students scoring <80 on the scenario were scheduled for a re-scenario. During the second year of scenarios, the faculty adapted and used a rubric as developed by Clark (2007) with her permission. Although course faculty reviewed the rubric at the beginning of the semester, new faculty were added to the course during the semester. Although the plan was for faculty to view videos of previous semester simulations to facilitate reliability, course and faculty issues prevented this necessary step, to our dismay. Therefore, faculty ($n = 6$) graded the scenarios inconsistently.

G. Debriefing Guidelines

A 10-minute debriefing follows each 20-minute scenario. The instructor begins with "What do you think you did well?" followed by "What would you like to do differently?" As part of the debriefing, students self-evaluate to identify their strengths and areas of concern from the simulation. Faculty facilitate and guide this conversation and assist with the identification of strategies to address problem areas.

H. & I. Suggestions/Key Features to Replicate or Improve

As students become more accustomed to simulation, these scenarios as developed may be used with junior-level students to teach and evaluate basic

20.1 Scenario Implementation: Initial Settings for Human Patient Simulator

CAPSTONE SCENARIO 1	CAPSTONE SCENARIO 2	CAPSTONE SCENARIO 3
Patient: Mrs. Edna Echo Monitor: Acute-care Setting	Patient: Mrs. Edna Echo Monitor: Acute-care Setting	Patient: Mrs. Edna Echo Monitor: Acute-care Setting

Initial State
Sinus rhythm: 97 bpm
Auscultation sounds:
   Left lung: Crackles
   Right lung: Crackles
   Bowel: Hypoactive
Airway: Reset all
Monitor controls:
   SpO_2: 94
   $etCO_2$: 34 mm Hg
   Tperi: 37.2°C
Respiration rate: 18 CO_2
Exhalation: Off
Blood pressure: 100/60
Handler:
   a. Nursing basics: Start
   b. IV start: Start
   c. Medication administration: Start
	Initial State
	Sinus rhythm: 97 bpm
	Auscultation sounds:
	   Left lung: Crackles
	   Right lung: Crackles
	   Bowel: Hypoactive
	Airway: Reset all
	Monitor controls:
	   SpO_2: 94
	   $etCO_2$: 34 mm Hg
	   Tperi: 37.2°C
	Respiration rate: 18 CO_2
	Exhalation: Off
	Blood pressure: 100/60
	Handler:
	   a. Nursing basics: Start
	   b. NG placement: Start
	   c. NG medication: Start
		Initial State
		Sinus rhythm: 98 bpm
		Auscultation sounds:
		   Left lung: Crackles
		   Right lung: Crackles
		   Bowel: Hypoactive
		Airway: Reset all
		Monitor controls:
		   SpO_2: 94
		   $etCO_2$: 34 mm Hg
		   Tperi: 37.2°C
		Respiration rate: 18 CO_2
		Exhalation: Off
		Blood pressure: 100/60
		Handler:
		   a. Nursing basics: Start
		   b. Medication administration (morphine): Start
		   c. Blood administration: Start

CAPSTONE SCENARIO 4	CAPSTONE SCENARIO 5	CAPSTONE SCENARIO 6
Patient: Mrs. Edna Echo Monitor: Acute-care Setting	Patient: Mrs. Edna Echo Monitor: Acute-care Setting	Patient: Mrs. Edna Echo Monitor: Acute-care Setting

Initial State
Sinus rhythm: 97 bpm
Auscultation sounds:
   Left lung: Crackles
   Right lung: Crackles
   Bowel: Hypoactive
Airway: Reset all
Monitor controls:
   SpO_2: = 94
   $etCO_2$: 34 mm Hg
   Tperi: 39.3°C
Respiration rate: 18 CO_2
Exhalation: Off
Blood pressure: 100/60
Handler:
   a. Nursing basics: Start
   b. IV piggyback: Start
   c. Trach suctioning: Start
	Initial State
	Sinus rhythm: 97 bpm
	Auscultation sounds:
	   Left lung: Crackles
	   Right lung: Crackles
	   Bowel: Hypoactive
	Airway: Reset all
	Monitor controls:
	   SpO_2: 94
	   $etCO_2$: 34 mm Hg
	   Tperi = 39.3°C
	Respiration rate: 18 CO_2
	Exhalation: Off
	Blood pressure: 100/60
	Handler:
	   a. Nursing basics: Start
	   b. Medication administration (morphine): Start
	   c. NG placement: Start
		Initial State
		Sinus rhythm: 109 bpm
		Auscultation sounds:
		   Left lung: Crackles
		   Right lung: Crackles
		   Bowel: Hypoactive
		Airway: Reset all
		Monitor controls:
		   SpO_2: = 92
		   $etCO_2$: = 34 mm Hg
		   Tperi: 40°C
		Respiration rate: 28 CO_2
		Exhalation: Off
		Blood pressure: 100/60
		Handler:
		   a. Nursing basics: Start
		   b. Isolation procedure: Start
		   c. Foley placement: Start

SpO_2, saturation of peripheral oxygen; $etCO_2$, end-tidal carbon dioxide; CO_2, carbon dioxide; NG, nasogastric.

nursing skills and communication techniques. In addition, more complexity can be added by including interdisciplinary roles. For example, a second nurse may be called to assist in the delivery of care or to notify a provider. As one of our College of Nursing graduate programs, nurse practitioner students may be a part of the simulations in the future, helping to hone their assessment skills and advanced-practice interventions.

Improvements to our senior simulations will include changes to grading and revision of our scenarios. As a result of the student evaluation inconsistencies, the plan is now that only two to three faculty will review three to five video simulations of past semesters using the rubric to establish beginning interrater reliability and then grade all scenarios in upcoming semesters. In addition, the rubric (Clark, 2007) will be further adapted with the author's permission, with the addition of safety, time management, organization, and critical thinking skills with examples. Our hope is then to establish interrater reliability by future testing with two external nursing universities at the approximate same stage of development in regard to simulations. Further changes include an increased emphasis on critical thinking. For example, in contrast to starting a blood transfusion as initially developed and implemented in our first year, now the student will work with a patient who has a blood transfusion in process who develops a blood transfusion reaction. Some of the previously used scenarios may be more appropriate for the junior-level students and are being shared with their faculty. This process will allow students to literally "build" on their knowledge, both cognitively and in psychomotor skills. Nursing "reports" at the beginning of scenarios will be shortened to minimize the student's focus on this content; report will be succinct, similar to a nursing report at change of shift. Patient information available through the "medical record" will be available but, as with the nursing report, much more concise. Student documentation will be more fully reviewed by faculty with the student, with particular emphasis on a focused patient assessment and legal safeguards. Lastly, an expectation is for the student to contact the provider by phone and report using Situation, Background, Recommendation, and Assessment (SBAR) with subsequent implementation of those orders.

J. Discussion of Simulation-Based Pedagogy and How This New Technology Has Contributed to Improved Student Outcomes

Students participating in simulations demonstrate an increased awareness of safety, organization, and time-management skills. In addition, there is an increased emphasis on critical-thinking skills. Written and verbal evaluative comments have included the increased stress associated with simulations as students choose and implement interventions without input from faculty, peers, or staff nurses. For many students, this is their first opportunity to demonstrate independence in the health care arena outside of their CIL practice sessions. Recent graduates who were in the first year of simulations speak of "I'm so glad we did that. It's just like what happens on the unit." Another comment frequently verbalized is, "I've had to make decisions on my own. It's scary but I'm glad it was with Mrs. Echo first." Faculty interested in simulation technology are considering the formation of a simulation research interest group to develop a program of research providing empirical evidence of change. The work has just begun. Our learning continues.

References

American Association of Colleges of Nursing. (2007). *The October 22, 2007 draft revision of the essentials of baccalaureate education for professional nursing practice.* Washington, DC: AACN.

Chambers, K. (2006). *Simulation experience evaluation tool.* Wappingers Falls, NY: Laerdal Medical Corporation.

Clark, M. (2007). *Clinical simulation grading rubric.* Unpublished master's thesis. Midwestern State University, Witchita Falls, Texas.

Haworth, J., & Conrad, C., (Eds.). (1996). Emblems of quality in higher education. In *Developing and sustaining high quality programs.* Boston: Allyn and Bacon.

National Council of State Boards of Nursing. (2007). *NCLEX-RN examination: Test plan for the national council licensure examination for registered nurses.* Retrieved June 18, 2008, from https://www.ncsbn.org/RN_Test_Plan_2007_Web.pdf

Recommended Reading and Resource

Joint Commission on Accreditation of Healthcare Organizations. (2006). Nurse's report to a physician. *Journal on Quality and Patient Safety, 32*(3), 172.

Laerdal Medical Corporation. (2007). *SimMan® Computer Software* (Version 3.3). Wappingers Falls, NY.

Improving Patient Safety Through Student Nurse–Resident Team Training: The Central Venous Catheterization Pilot Project

21

Laura T. Gantt,
Walter C. Robey III,
Tamara L. Congdon,
and Linda Bolin

A. Discussion of Implementation of Simulation-Based Pedagogy in Each Contributor's Individualized Teaching

Central venous catheterization is a high-risk, invasive procedure with the potential for adverse events. In 2007, the Central Venous Catheterization (CVC) Quality and Safety Initiative was instituted as a collaboration between the Brody School of Medicine (BSOM) at East Carolina University and Pitt County Memorial Hospital (PCMH) in Greenville, North Carolina. The goal of the initiative was to decrease the number of infections and adverse mechanical events associated with the procedure by providing first-year resident physicians with standardized, simulation-based training in central line placement. This successful program is currently in its second year.

The Medical Simulation and Patient Safety Laboratory (MSPSL) at BSOM played a central role in the development of the CVC initiative. The MSPSL originated within the Department of Emergency Medicine (EM) and has now grown to include a number of components. These include a series of hands-on emergency skills workshops, an advanced invasive procedures lab, a gross anatomy lab, technical skills training using task trainers and inanimate models, and the high-fidelity Emergency Care Simulator Lab. Standardized patients and trained actors are integrated into educational simulations. The lab also has the ability to produce instructional videography.

Until recently, resident physicians have been trained independent of other disciplines in CVC within the MSPSL. In 2006, when the East Carolina University College of Nursing (CON) moved to its current location close to BSOM and PCMH, new opportunities for joint efforts between the academic and patient care organizations presented themselves. In this pilot project, a CVC-trained team consisting of a resident physician from BSOM and a senior student nurse from CON was created with the ultimate goal of improving patient safety during the performance of this invasive procedure in a simulated environment. This project represents one of the first collaborations between faculties of the BSOM and the CON.

Due to the fact that the CVC initiative began prior to the decision to embark on this pilot project, the objectives for the course, which were developed 2 years ago, remained essentially the same for this pilot. The learning and scenario objectives for physicians in the CVC course were as follows:

- Develop a working knowledge of CVC and how to recognize and minimize adverse patient events associated with the procedure;
- Learn how to safely perform CVC.

The director of the MSPSL approached the director of the CON labs about the pilot project after working with and looking at videos of the residents performing CVC in simulated environments. What the MSPSL director recognized was that in the actual patient care environment, physicians would usually require and receive assistance during the CVC procedure from registered nurses. Undergraduate senior student nurses were believed to be the best level of students to participate in the project because of their mastery of previous course content around anatomy and physiology, communication, and medical asepsis. First-semester senior-level students are in predictable clinical rotations that make their recruitment for projects, such as this one, more feasible. CON course coordinator and department chair approval was obtained, as was an IRB exemption for educational research.

B. Description of Educational Materials Available in Your Teaching Area and Relative to Your Specialty

The objectives for the clinical component of the first semester senior nursing course are as follows:

- Apply theories, concepts, scientific principles, and professional standards to implement a holistic plan of care for clients experiencing complex alterations in health.
- Use critical thinking and scientific reasoning to implement therapeutic nursing interventions in the care of adults with complex alterations in health.

■ Collaborate with interdisciplinary teams to develop strategies that promote health, maximize quality of life, and maintain optimal functioning,
including care at the end of life.
■ Demonstrate professional behaviors while providing safe, therapeutic
nursing care with diverse clients in a variety of settings.
■ Collaborate with interdisciplinary teams, clients, and families in the
client's transition across health care settings.

These course objectives were in line with faculty goals for this pilot.

For student nurses, the American Association of Colleges of Nursing's *Essentials of Baccalaureate Education for Professional Nursing Practice* (AACN, 2007)
addressed by course and scenario objectives are as follows:

Essential II: Basic Organizational and Systems Leadership for Quality Care
Essential VI: Interprofessional Communication and Collaboration for Im-
proving Health Care Outcomes
Essential VIII: Professionalism and Professional Values
Essential IX: Baccalaureate Generalist Nursing Practice

For all scenarios, the National Council of State Boards of Nursing *National
Council Licensure Examination for Registered Nurses* (NCSBN-RN) test plan categories and subcategories (NCSBN, 2007) addressed are as follows:

Safe, Effective Care Environment
    Management of Care
        Establishing Priorities
        Performance Improvement (Quality Improvement)
        Collaboration with Interdisciplinary Team
        Informed Consent
    Safety and Infection Control
        Standard/Transmission-Based/Other Precautions
        Medical and Surgical Asepsis
        Safe Use of Equipment
        Error Prevention
Physiological Integrity
    Basic Care and Comfort
        Non-pharmacological Comfort Interventions
    Pharmacological and Parenteral Therapies
        Adverse Effects/Contraindications
        Expected Effects/ Outcomes
        Central Venous Access Devices
        Parenteral/Intravenous Therapies
    Reduction of Risk Potential
        Vital Signs
        System Specific Assessments
    Physiological Adaptation
        Unexpected Response to Therapies
        Hemodynamics

Description of Participants

Four emergency medicine residents and four senior student nurses were recruited to participate in the pilot study. Both groups completed a Web-based CVC training module (Kaye & Grant, n.d.) with pre- and posttesting. This training module took each learner approximately 3 hours to complete. Prior to the beginning of the training, the CON faculty developed a student nurse CVC checklist, with specific roles for the student nurses. The checklist (see below) was discussed at a clinical conference prior to the training with a session to familiarize learners with the CVC tray and to review sterile technique.

ECU Student Nurse and CVC Project

Checklist for Undergraduate Student Nurses in CVC Scenarios

Preparation for Scenarios

_____1. Review basic Anatomy and Physiology text: Central vs. peripheral veins and anatomical landmarks.

_____2. View Duke University online CVC program: Complete pre- and posttest.

_____3. Review Fundamentals text: Preparing patient for procedure and sterile technique.

_____4. Review Medical-Surgical text: Caring for complex patient requiring CVC.

_____5. Familiarize yourself with CVC kits.

_____6. Perform literature search on CVC as related to nursing care: Submit one article with brief review of article.

Responsibilities on Day of Scenario:

_____1. Review medical chart to check for allergies and orders (IV fluids).

_____2. Set up IV infusion according to orders.

_____3. Gather necessary equipment/supplies.

_____4. Assist with setting up room with input from CVC team.

_____5. Position equipment (ultrasound [US] machine) and supplies (CVC tray) appropriately in room based on provider preference and patient situation.

_____6. Communicate with CVC team (re: student nurse vs. medical provider responsibilities).

_____7. Introduce self to patient on entering room.

_____8. Position patient appropriately.

_____9. Connect patient to monitor, and assure equipment is working properly.

_____10. Reiterate procedure to patient and student nurse's role during procedure.

_____11. Assist provider with setting up sterile CVC tray prn.

_____12. Assist provider with gowning procedure prn.

_____13. Observe/anticipate methods to maintain sterile technique.

_____14. Communicate and offer reassurance to patient throughout procedure.

_____15. Respond to the needs of the provider during the procedure (e.g., extra equipment needs, changing the patient's position).

_____16. Observe monitor and patient's status throughout the procedure.

_____17. Dispose of sharps properly after insertion completed and clean up prn.

_____18. Remove sterile drape, and communicate to patient that procedure is done.

_____19. Ensure CVC disc and kit are applied according to hospital protocol.

_____20. Ensure chest x-ray (CXR) ordered and final report received prior to infusing IV fluids.

_____21. Reposition patient.

_____22. Document procedure.

C. Describe Running of the Scenario

On the day of the pilot, nursing students rotated through sequential skills stations taught by BSOM faculty and upper-level emergency medicine residents. Small group instruction with residents and nursing students focused on team dynamics, communication, sterile and procedural technique, and patient monitoring using a combination of simulation modalities. The skills stations, which took approximately 3 to 4 hours at the beginning of the day, were comparable to the initial "resident only" CVC training.

Skills station 1 uses a patient actor needing central venous access. The resident and/or student nurse will do the following:

- Discuss indications for the CVC.
- Obtain or assist in obtaining informed consent.
- Prepare the patient for the procedure.
- Identify anatomical landmarks.
- Identify vascular structures using ultrasound (US).
- Practice sterile preparation and aseptic technique, including US-guided sterile technique.

Skills station 2 uses a simple Seldinger wire technique task trainer. The resident and/or student nurse will do the following:

- Review the CVC tray components.
- Practice the Seldinger wire technique.

Skills station 3 uses task trainers to practice cannulation vessels. The resident and/or student nurse will do the following:

- Practice intrajugular and subclavian vessel catheterization using an anatomic approach on the Laerdal torso.
- Practice intrajugular vessel catheterization using US guidance on the Simulab CentraLineMan.

The faculties of CON and BSOM elected not to alter the components of the course significantly for purposes of the pilot. The CVC course content addresses varied learning styles through online didactic, task-training, skills-station, and high-fidelity simulation components. Both faculties believed that the course offered a good opportunity for the student nurses and some of the residents to interact and that the common knowledge gained in the course would contribute to team members being "on the same page" during the scenarios.

Random student nurse–resident team assignments were made. The teams were scheduled for scenarios with videotaping immediately following the skills stations. For the student nurses, this pilot counted the equivalent of a 9-hour clinical day and took the place of an alternate clinical observation day.

D. Presentation of Completed Template

Title: Central Venous Line Insertion and Care by Student Nurse–Resident Teams

Level:
First-semester senior BSN students and first- and second-year emergency medicine residents

Focus Area:
Inpatient and/or emergency care

Scenario Description:
What follows is a copy of the chart information assembled for this scenario:

EAST CAROLINA UNIVERSITY SCHOOL OF NURSING
VIRTUAL HOSPITAL

Greenville, North Carolina

Physician Progress Note

Patient Name: Gordon, Walter	**MR#:** CAR-024
Date of Birth: 2/15/50	**Age:** 57 years
Address: Anywhere, USA 23970	**Code Status:** Full Code
Phone: cell 252-900-WINN	**Religion:** Christian
Family: Gordon, Jeff (son)	**Occupation:** Race car driver
Allergies: No known allergies	

Today @ 0015. 57-year-old Native American male brought to Emergency Room by local ambulance at 0015. Patient presented with severe dyspnea and dehydration. Unremarkable medical history. No mental health history. No surgeries. No known allergies to medications, food, or environment. Height: 5' 8", 178 lb. Current medications: Daily vitamins only; no alcohol, no cigarettes or recreational drugs.

Good social and family support. Patient reports private insurance, denies financial concerns. Patient indicated sick for several days with "bad cold." On admission, pulse ox 88%. Minimal respiratory distress. Placed on O_2 @ 2 L / NC, with improved saturation 95%. Chest x-ray, labs, IV initiated. Admitted ICU.

Admitting Diagnosis: Pneumonia, fever, dehydration

Electronic Signature: Dr. OnCall, # 3908

Today @ 0315. Some improvement in respiratory status, but IV infiltration. No IV access. Discussed and reviewed options for central line placement. Informed consent obtained for central line for antibiotic use by patient and son. All in agreement and consent signed.

Electronic Signature: Dr. OnCall, # 3908

Setting the Scene:

> *Equipment needed:*
> - Simulator (SimMan®) with gown, identification band, and gender-appropriate body parts
> - Microphone or other device to allow communication between learners and simulator operator
> - Audio-video recording device
> - Medical equipment: Patient monitor, pulse oximeter, blood pressure cuff, oxygen hook-up and flow meter, suction with canister and tubing for low wall suction, stethoscope, US machine
> - Sink for hand washing and/or waterless hand cleaner
> - Medical supply cart with supplies, including CVC trays, sterile gowns, masks, sterile and nonsterile gloves.
>
> *Medical record:*
> - Patient chart to include progress notes and patient consent
>
> *Resources needed:*
> - CVC policy and procedure, procedure checklist
>
> *Participants needed:*
> - student nurse, 1 emergency medicine resident, 1 simulator operator (staff, faculty, or instructional technology personnel), 1 faculty observer/evaluator, 1 videographer

Scenario Implementation:

Initial Settings for Human Patient Simulator

- Temp: 40°C
- Heart rate/Rhythm: Normal sinus at 109 bpm
- Respiratory rate: 28
- SpO$_2$: 95%
- Lungs sounds: Crackles in both lungs
- BP: 100/60

At the end of the scenario, each student nurse documented the care they provided to the "patient."

Evaluative Criteria:

Our goal as faculty members was to provide as much training and support in advance of the simulation as possible and then not to interfere with the simulation once it began. Student nurse–resident teams worked through procedural or communication problems as they developed. Faculty assisted only when asked and functioned in the role of nursing assistant or unlicensed assistive personnel. Simulations were video recorded for review and scoring. Teams were evaluated during simulated performance of a CVC insertion. Additional evaluation took place during viewing of videotapes after the simulations.

Nurse and physician faculty piloted a variety of tools to evaluate the residents and nursing students during the pilot. For *team training components*, the Mayo High Performance Teamwork Scale (Malec et al., 2007) was used to rate each team; the scale has established reliability and validity. Participants completed a *self-assessment* using this same scale related to team impact on their performance. *Technical skills* were evaluated using task-specific checklists developed for the project. *Learner satisfaction* with this educational experience was individually evaluated using a satisfaction survey (Chambers, 2006) previously used in CON as well as one developed at BSOM for this project.

Data analysis is ongoing at this time. Based on team member and simulation experience evaluations, residents and student nurses uniformly found the team scenario to have been worthwhile. The residents, who had completed a similar scenario in a simulation environment with less fidelity and without the student nurses, noted how valuable the student nurses were in assisting with the placement of the CVC; residents noted an increase in their ability to maintain sterility and proper technique. The student nurses valued the opportunity to work *with* another health science discipline as an alternative to the parallel process that often occurs in the education of various health care team members; they were able to help monitor and respond to the "patient" in the simulated environment. The addition of a trained student nurse to assist during the procedure provided students and residents an opportunity to synthesize and apply technical skills and clinical judgment to improve quality outcomes and safety for the patient. The student nurses, who will be evaluated using simulation scenarios in their final semester before graduation, appreciated this additional opportunity to practice live scenarios.

During the CON faculty debriefing of the student nurses, the group discussed team dynamics and reflected on previously undefined issues that may affect team members and patient care situations. At the completion of the pilot, CON faculty reviewed the student nurse responsibilities during the scenario and found that the students successfully completed 70% to 87% of items on the checklist. Of those items on the checklist deemed "critical" by CON faculty, the students completed between 57% and 66%. These findings have implications for how this content is taught in the future.

Videos of student nurse–resident CVC teams were individually viewed and scored by CON and BSOM faculty utilizing the Mayo High Performance Teamwork Scale (MHPTS). The independent scoring allowed for decreased bias by limiting discussions during the scoring. This was our first opportunity to use the MHPTS. The scale is easy to use and requires little training.

E. Recommendations for Further Use

In reviewing the results to date, the combined faculties have identified a number of improvements that should be made if the project should be replicated. First and foremost, this pilot took a great deal more time and human resources to plan and implement than was expected. Identifying dates when CON and BSOM faculty, residents, and student nurses could be in the labs together was extremely challenging. Ultimately, time constraints affected all other aspects of the project.

Objectives for the CVC team training course and scenarios need to be further developed separately from other related courses. The faculty did not think to do this until well into the project. The scenario was not scripted but was run "live." The advantage to this is that there was flexibility in "patient" responses based on student nurse and resident actions; the disadvantage is that there was inconsistency in the running of the scenario, which detracted from our ability to compare the performance of the teams.

Group and team prebriefing with orientation to course objectives and associated checklists and scales did not occur in the pilot. The student nurses were debriefed as a group a week after the scenarios. Group resident and student nurse–resident team debriefings are pending.

In the future, however, raters will meet to discuss scale components in advance of evaluation to ensure consistency in rating. The MHPTS lacks a comments section; in reviewing the results, raters had frequently written in the margins. In discussions between CON and BSOM faculties, it was discovered that a checklist or other tool, like the one developed for the student nurses, was needed to accompany the MHPTS to help identify individual performance issues that affected team performance.

The addition of a trained student nurse to assist during this high-risk invasive procedure provided students and residents an opportunity to synthesize and apply technical skills and clinical judgment to improve quality outcomes and safety for the patient.

References

American Association of Colleges of Nursing. (2007). *The October 22, 2007 draft revision of the essentials of baccalaureate education for professional nursing practice.* Washington, DC: AACN.

Chambers, K. (2006). *Simulation experience evaluation tool.* Wappingers Falls, NY: Laerdal Medical Corporation.

Kaye, K., & Grant, J. (n.d.). *Insertion of central venous catheters.* Retrieved November 7, 2007, from http://cvctraining.medicine.duke.edu

Malec, J., Torsher, L., Dunn, W., Wiegmann, D., Arnold, J., Brown, D., et al. (2007). The Mayo high performance teamwork scale: Reliability and validity for evaluating key crew resource management skill. *Simulation in Healthcare, 2*(1), 4–10.

National Council of State Boards of Nursing. (2007). *NCLEX-RN examination: Test plan for the National Council Licensure Examination for Registered Nurses.* Retrieved June 18, 2008, from https://www.ncsbn.org/RN_Test_Plan_2007_Web.pdf

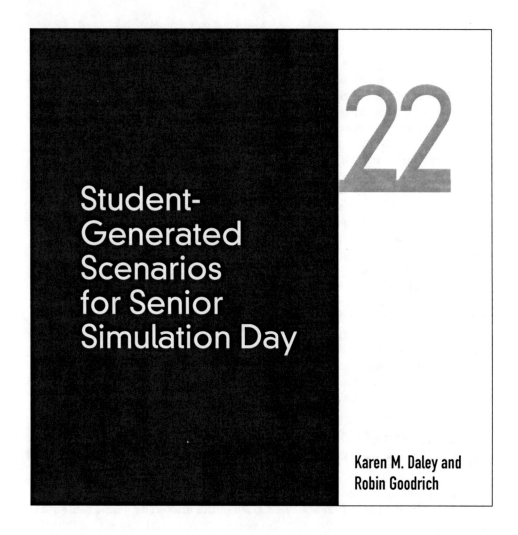

22

Student-Generated Scenarios for Senior Simulation Day

Karen M. Daley and Robin Goodrich

A. Discussion of Implementation of Simulation-Based Pedagogy in Each Contributor's Individualized Teaching

Implementation of simulation-based pedagogy has progressed rapidly at Western Connecticut State University over the past 5 years. Initially, all simulations were done on static manikins and were primarily skill based. As the lead instructors in the capstone course in the spring semester of 2008, we felt it very important to expose senior students to high-fidelity simulation. High-fidelity simulation allows the student to link theory, utilize the nursing process, and apply curricular content using a multidisciplinary approach. Additional advantages of high-fidelity simulation include enhancement of psychomotor skills and collaboration with peers and faculty in a nonthreatening environment.

Obtaining our first human patient simulator (HPS) took several tries and much effort over a 2-year period. Once obtained, we made it an immediate priority to introduce high-fidelity simulations at the senior level. This effort turned out to be extremely timely. That year, one of the regional hospitals began competency testing using the HPS. Our graduates, it was reported, were some of the only new graduates that excelled in the testing.

As time has gone by, we have introduced simulation at all levels of our program. By the time the seniors arrive in the capstone course, they have become accustomed to interacting with the HPS and have developed their own "simulation personalities." For instance, some come hungry for as much simulation as possible. Others have arrived and announced that they have done so much simulation, they are "sick and tired of it!" This year, the students arrived and stated they had not done enough simulation and were asking for dedicated time in a nontesting situation to reacquaint themselves with the HPS. As with all capstone courses, our job as faculty is to assess each group's final learning needs and meet them in the best way we see fit. However, this year we have found that the capstone course itself was so anxiety producing that testing on the simulators did not seem feasible. In fact, once the students had completed their intensive capstone course clinical, assessing competencies was not an issue.

Encouraging and supporting critical thinking is, however, a continuous challenge, and simulations serve as a fun yet challenging way to work to synthesize all that has been learned throughout the program as well as within the capstone course. Larew, Lessans, Spunt, Foster, and Covington (2005) suggest that groups of students be asked to develop scenarios as an experiential learning exercise. As a result, this year, we have introduced a "Senior Simulation Day" as a substitution for a clinical day to meet the needs of this group of seniors in which seniors were asked to create student-generated scenarios.

B. Description of Educational Materials Available in Your Teaching Area and Relative to Your Specialty

Simulation facilities have more than tripled in the Nursing Department in the last 5 years. In academic year 2002–2003, when the university held a centennial celebration, nursing graduates from 30 years ago returned and stated that the nursing labs had remained "much the same" as when they were students. Since then, the Nursing Department has worked tirelessly to upgrade and renovate the original nursing lab and expand the facilities to now include three nursing labs, with a fourth ICU lab opening in fall 2008. Each of these labs house an HPS with a designated area and equipment for use with that HPS. In addition, we have found that a student resource center with textbooks, a seminar table, and references is essential for debriefing, processing, and re-do planning of scenarios. Students have access to online resources and drug references as well as the entire lab. Currently, we do not have the space or facilities for using a control room for simulations, so we have upgraded to remote personal digital assistant (PDA) access for instructors who would like to run the scenarios remotely from the HPS. Often, these scenarios are run by only one instructor, and having a scenario control person is often not possible.

C. Specific Objective for Simulation Utilization Within a Specific Course and the Overall Program

Our objective is to test senior nursing students' basic program outcome competencies and knowledge synthesis through creation of one simulated scenario of an advanced medical-surgical disease/condition, integrating the nursing process, communication skills, nursing skills, and critical thinking. Students then try to "stump" their classmates by testing the observing group's knowledge of the medical-surgical problem.

D. Introduction of Scenario to Include Setting the Scene, Technology Used, Objectives, and Description of Participants

Students are instructed to "mock up" a high-fidelity HPS to make the scenario as real as possible. They are given full access to the Medical-Surgical Lab and are allowed to use any equipment they need from the lab supplies, including IVs, IV machines, and Foley catheters.

Objectives

Students will be able to identify a common medical-surgical problem from their recent clinical experiences and create a scenario that allows the following:

- Portrays assessment factors and vital statistics common to that problem.
- Utilizes a chart and medication record with the appropriate drugs and dosages for that disease.
- Shows common psychosocial issues and concerns through communication with the patients, health care providers, and significant others.
- Requires interventions and evaluations appropriate to the standard of care for the medical-surgical problem being covered that result, through the playing out of the scenario, in an improvement in the patient's condition.

The National Council of State Boards of Nursing's *National Council Licensure Examination for Registered Nurses* (NCLEX-RN) test plan categories and subcategories (NCSBN, 2007) addressed in the simulation are as follows:

Safe and Effective Care Environment
    Management of Care
        Collaboration with Interdisciplinary Team
        Delegation
        Establishing Priorities
        Ethical Practice
        Informed Consent
        Legal Rights and Responsibilities
        Resource Management
    Safety and Infection Control
        Medical and Surgical Asepsis

        Safe Use of Equipment
        Standard/Transmission-Based/Other Precautions
    Health Promotion and Maintenance
        Family Systems
        Techniques of Physical Assessment
    Psychosocial Integrity
        Coping Mechanisms
        Therapeutic Communications
        Unexpected Body Image Changes
    Physiological Integrity
      Basic Care and Comfort
        Elimination
        Non-Pharmacological Comfort Interventions
        Personal Hygiene
        Rest and sleep
      Pharmacological and Parenteral Therapy
        Dosage Calculation
        Expected Effects/Outcomes
        Medication Administration
        Parenteral/Intravenous Therapies
        Pharmacological Agents/Actions
        Pharmacological Pain Management
      Reduction of Risk Potential
        Diagnostic Tests
        Laboratory Values
        Potential for Complications of Diagnostic Tests/Treatments/
          Procedures
        System Specific Assessments
        Therapeutic Procedures
        Vital Signs
      Physiological Adaptation
        Hemodynamics
        Illness Management
        Medical Emergencies

Description of Participants

We encouraged all students in the group who create each scenario to become involved in the scenario. One student is the scenario controller and runs the computer or PDA as the scenario progresses. The HPS is the patient, and the other students may become the wife, doctor, nurse, or other participants at the discretion of the student creators.

E. Describe Running of the Scenario

Students are instructed to access the following simulation assignment from the course Web site 1 week prior to the simulation day:

NUR 375 Nursing Practicum

Senior Simulation Day

This day is designed to refamiliarize you with the HPS SimMan®. Many hospitals now test basic nursing competencies of new graduates in orientation with the SimMan®. Today, we will be creating scenarios from your experience or your imagination. We will split the group in two, and one group will test the other on an advanced medical-surgical scenario.

Objective: To test senior nursing students on one advanced medical-surgical disease/condition, integrating the nursing process, communication skills, nursing skills, and critical thinking.

E-Res resource: Under "daley" on E-Res you will find the NURSIM E-Res site.

(1) Print out the Laerdal Scenario Planning Worksheet (Laerdal Medical, 2008a)(first two pages only) and the Scenario Validation Sheet (Laerdal Medical, 2008b) and bring them to clinical on Simulation Day.
(2) View the SimMan® Introduction PowerPoint about simulation and SimMan®.
(3) Feel free to browse other documents or links. If you want to know more about the computers hiding in SimMan® and the setup, you can look at the SimMan®/SimBaby® PowerPoint (we do not have SimBaby® yet).

Assignment:

- Design a medical-surgical scenario based on a real patient or a simulated patient to run for another group of students as if you are the instructor.
- You will need to mock up SimMan® to look as "real" as possible. You can use any equipment in the WH Nursing Lab; for example, IVs, the IV machine, medication, carts, Foleys, etc.
- You may decide to use other students as actors; for example, the distraught wife, the rude doctor, the inattentive nurse
- Write out how the scenario will progress on the second page of the planning sheet. Include dialog, SimMan® settings (RR, P, BP, pulse oximeter, etc.), and equipment needed. Include all the knowledge you want to test on the crucial aspects of the disease/condition and meds. List all nursing assessment and interventions needed in order for the patient to improve.
- Just like a play, all scenarios have a beginning, middle, and end, so don't forget to plan for an ending (e.g., the patient with difficulty breathing is breathing better). But, scenarios often take on a life of their own, so limit to 15 minutes.

Good luck and have fun!

Prior to arriving for the simulation day, students should download and print the scenario template and evaluation criteria. Students are also instructed to brainstorm on their own about comprehensive scenarios that test in-depth knowledge about common problems they encountered in the capstone clinical. Students are instructed that to produce a chart, medication sheet, and history for their simulated patient, keeping in mind that they will need to construct the scenario much as they would write a play. On Senior Simulation Day, faculty introduce each group to the simulation technology from the instructor side. Faculty demonstrate simulation technology and the features of the HPS to the student groups. Students are expected to run the scenario themselves in its entirety. Faculty support is available, although independence of the group is encouraged.

F. Presentation of Completed Template

A total of 37 students in five clinical groups were given this assignment. The capstone course coordinator, who is the resident expert on simulation, attended all simulation events along with the clinical instructors. A total of six scenarios were created by the students. Three are presented here. In the end, only four clinical groups participated due to timing issues and scheduling (maternity leave, family emergencies, and illness). Those not participating were given an alternate assignment.

Sample Student-Generated Senior Scenarios 1–3

Scenario #1

Title: Joe Money
Nursing 375, Nursing Practicum

Focus Area:
Senior scenario

Scenario Description:
Joe Money is a 59-year-old man found on the scene unresponsive with a BP of 180/90, weak thready pulses, no reflexes, flaccid extremities, fixed pinpoint pupils, and a history of drug and alcohol (ETOH) abuse. Transported to the emergency room, where his BP is now 230/108, with severe respiratory depression progressing to apnea. Patient may also have a head trauma and increased intracranial pressure. When his clothes are removed, $800, a switchblade, and a syringe are found in his jean pockets.

Scenario Objectives:

1. Demonstrates proper assessment for drug overdose and trauma with appropriate interventions, including assessment of airway, breathing, and circulation (ABCs).
2. Performs assessment and interventions for increased intracranial pressure.
3. Staff uses proper safety precautions for potential drug abuse patients.

Setting the Scene:

> *Equipment needed:* HPS, patient monitor, O_2 hookup, pulse oximeter, blood pressure cuff, stethoscope, paper chart for documentation, syringe, money, fake switchblade, 2 large bore IVs, IV machine, Foley catheter, several vials of mock IV push drugs and IV access syringes.
> *Resources needed:* Textbooks, drug books, computer access

Simulator level: High fidelity

Participants needed:

Student to run the computer for the HPS

Scene 1: Drug user and a student to play Joe Money, two students to play EMTs who transport the patient

Scene 2: HPS plays Joe Money, two students play emergency room nurses

Scenario Implementation:

Initial scene takes place in an apartment as the patient sells drugs to a customer and then sits down to drink alcohol and smoke crack cocaine. Patient passes out, and EMTs are called.

Scenario resumes in the Emergency Room, where the patient is now played by the HPS. Two emergency room nurses are assessing the patient and reporting the results to the observing students, who are making suggestions and recommendations for care. Students use the nursing process as a guiding framework for moving through the scenario.

Initial settings for HPS: BP 180/90 at the scene then 230/108 in the emergency room. Variable bradycardia with irregular beat, shallow and slow respirations of 5 to 10 progressing to Cheyne-Stokes and then apnea. EKG shows a bundle branch block typical of cocaine abuse. Emergency room nurse (played by student) reports weak thready pulse; toxicology screen positive for cocaine and high blood alcohols levels; and blood gases of PCO2 32, pH 7.54, PO2 47, Na 147, and glucose 181. Results of CT scan show multiple bilateral deep and superficial cerebral hematomas.

Required Student Assessments and Actions

_____ Identify symptoms of respiratory depression and cardiac abnormality.

_____ Initiate two large-bore IVs.

_____ Suggest C-spine x-ray, CT scan, and ABGs based on assessment findings and history.

_____ Raise head of the bed secondary to increasing intracranial pressure.

_____ Assess blood tests, toxicology screen, and urinalysis.

_____ Insert Foley, and assess drainage of 3,000 cc over an hour as sign of diabetes insipidus/increasing intracranial pressure.

_____ Obtain EKG, and recognize bundle branch block as a sign of cocaine abuse.

_____ Administer medications prescribed. Check dosages and five rights.

_____ Assess results of x-rays and ABGs, and recommend actions.

_____ Suggest airlift transport to a Level I trauma hospital once stabilized.

Evaluative Criteria:

_____ Students who have created the scenario use the nursing process to cue the observing students to make recommendations about patient care. Cues are adequate for recognition by the observing students.

_____ Students observing were able to recognize signs and symptoms as drug and alcohol overdose and proceed with appropriate interventions and safety precautions.

_____ Students observing were able to recognize the signs and symptoms of possible trauma and follow diagnostic protocol to assess and begin interventions for trauma and increasing intracranial pressure.

_____ Students observing were able to connect the cardiac arrhythmia with the patient's drug abuse.

_____ Student observing were able to accurately assess abnormal blood gases and suggest treatment.

_____ Students observing were able to suggest correct medication and dosages to treat patient's condition.

_____ Patient stabilizes enough for transport, but students watch for signs of impending herniation and possible negative outcome.

Scenario #2

Title: Addison Jane
Nursing 375, Nursing Practicum

Focus Area:
Senior scenario

Scenario Description:
Addison Jane is a 62-year-old white female with a history of hypertension and hyperlipidemia who was found in her driveway near gardening tools by a bystander clutching her chest and appearing pale. In addition, she has blood on her right earlobe. Patient weighs 165 lb and is allergic to aspirin and penicillin. Her medications are unknown. Pregnant daughter is called and is nearby in the Emergency Room.

Scenario Objectives:

1. Uses initial assessment/focused history when evaluating patient.
2. Prioritizes and initiates emergency patient care with stabilization of the cervical spine.
3. Performs automated external defibrillator.
4. Understands how to clear patient during the delivery of shocks in defibrillation.
5. Demonstrates assessment of patient's response to resuscitation.
6. Properly documents events during the emergency care.

Setting the Scene:

Equipment needed: HPS, patient monitor, O_2 hook-up, bandages, pulse oximeter, blood pressure cuff, stethoscope, paper chart

Resources needed: Textbooks, computer access for database search and evidence-based practice

Simulator level: High fidelity

Participants needed: Two nurses, doctor who yells incorrect orders, pregnant family member whose water breaks in the middle of the code, student to run the computer for the HPS

Scenario Implementation:

Initial settings for the HPS include HR: 62, BP: 106/72, RR: 12, pulse oximeter: 94%

Required Student Assessments and Actions

_____ Perform initial assessment and cervical spine immobilization.

_____ Perform EKG, and recognize deterioration to ventricular fibrillation with
no BP and HR of <140.

_____ Correctly perform CPR with the use of a bag-valve mask.

_____ Apply automated electronic defibrillator (AED).

_____ Administer three shocks at the correct setting despite physician giving
incorrect orders.

_____ Perform CPR.

_____ Establish IV access.

_____ Gives medications as appropriate: Epinephrine q 3–5 minutes; atropine
q 3–5 minutes

_____ Patient response to interventions: return to bradycardic sinus rhythm
with vital signs of BP 85/52, P 34, O_2 88%, with weak thready pulse and
normal heart sounds.

_____ Interventions continue with re-medication of atropine and the addition
of amiodarone with improvement of vital signs to BP 104/68, P 65, and
O_2 94%.

_____ Once stabilized, patient is recommended to be sent for head-neck evaluation and MRI.

Evaluative Criteria:

_____ Correct interventions result in stabilization of the patient.

_____ Students who have created the scenario use the nursing process to cue the
observing students to make recommendations about patient care. Cues
are adequate for recognition by the observing students.

_____ Students observing were able to recognize signs and symptoms of possible trauma and severe hypovolemia.

_____ Students observing are able to follow proper protocol in directing the
sequence of CPR.

_____ Students take proper safety precautions.

Scenario #3

Title: Dolly
Nursing 375, Nursing Practicum

Focus Area:
Senior scenario

Scenario Description:
Dolly is a 45-year-old woman admitted with a MRSA infection of a wound. Her
temperature at home was 102°F, with complaints of overall achiness, loss of
appetite, and diaphoresis. She has a past medical history of type II diabetes,

hypertension, increased cholesterol blood levels, and depression. Wound is currently a stage 3 in the lumbar sacral area. She weighs 325 lb and is 5′ 4″ tall.

Scenario Objectives:

1. Students will be able to state some orders a doctor would write for the signs and symptoms observed.
2. Students will be able to state five continuous orders for a patients with a suspected pulmonary embolism.
3. Students will be able to state five discharge orders for someone recovering from a pulmonary embolism.

Setting the Scene:

> *Equipment needed:* HPS, patient monitor, O_2 hookup, bandages, pulse oximeter, blood pressure cuff, stethoscope, paper chart, thermometer, nasal cannula, IV machine, IV bag with vancomycin and IV bag with heparin and secondary line, primary line
>
> *Resources needed:* Textbooks, computer access for database search and evidence-based practice
>
> *Simulator level:* High fidelity
>
> *Participants needed:* Uninterested RN, patient technician, medical doctor.

Scenario Implementation:

> Initial settings for HPS include BP: 130/70, P: 72, RR: 12, T: 102°F.
>
> *Day #1 in emergency room:* Complaining of decreased appetite, and not feeling well. Found to have a fever of 102°F and a stage 3 lumbar sacral ulcer. After culture, the wound is found to be infected with MRSA. Patient admitted to the floor with an IV infusion of vancomycin.
>
> *Day #3 on the patient floor:*
>
> **0800:** WBC 1,300, no c/o of pain, BP 130/72, P 85, Temp 99.2°F, O_2 98% on RA. Patient refuses to get out of bed since admission. Only uses bedpan.
>
> **1200:** Patient care technician comes in for vital signs and reports to the RN: BP 130/79, RR 26, P 120, Temp 100.2°F, O_2 94% on RA. Patient states "My chest hurts, and I can't breathe." RN seems uninterested in patient and states she is going on break and will check on patient after her break. Tells patient care technician to keep an eye on the patient.
>
> **1300:** RN finally gets around to assessing patient and finds wheezes, 7/10 substernal chest pain. Nonproductive cough and increased anxiety. O_2 has dropped to 86%, and pulse is 130.
>
> RN puts oxygen on patient 2 L nasal cannula, and O_2 comes up to 90%
>
> RN proceeds to call MD, who orders EKG, cardiac enzymes, chest x-ray (CXR) and 1 mg morphine IV.
>
> **1400:** Results:
>
> *EKG:* Sinus tachycardia
>
> *Cardiac enzymes:* Negative
>
> *CXR:* Infiltrates, elevated diaphragm on right side. Doctor suspects pulmonary embolism (PE) and orders baseline coagulation studies: PT, PTT,

and INR; spiral CT to verify PE; heparin bolus 10,000 U and maintenance 1,600 U per hour.

1500: Vital signs as follows: BP 120/70, RR 20, P 100, Temp 99.0°F, O_2 97% on 2 L NC. Pain level 5/10 and given 1 mg morphine IV

MD continuous orders: High Fowler, incentive spirometer every 2 hours, out of bed as soon as possible with the assistance of physical therapy. Thromboguards, monitor blood values especially PT, INR.

Day # 7 Discharge

MD discharge instructions: Decrease weight, take Coumadin as prescribed, TED stockings, visiting nurses, active range of motion to all extremities, out of bed as much as tolerated, do not dangle or cross legs

Required Student Assessments and Actions

_____ Students in scenario assess and intervene in the emergency room based on the recommendations of observing students.

    _____ Assess VS, wound, and do a focused assessment/history of patient.

    _____ Obtain IV access and begin antibiotic therapy.

    _____ Transfer to floor with orders.

_____ Assessment of vital signs on Day 3 by RN.

_____ Evaluation of assessment data by RN and interventions at the bedside by administering O_2.

_____ Use of SBAR format in communication with MD.

_____ Order and obtain required blood and diagnostic tests.

_____ Evaluate blood tests and communicate with MD.

_____ Set up and administer heparin as ordered.

_____ Interact appropriately with patient to explain new orders.

_____ Delegate appropriate interventions to patient care technician. Communicate clearly.

_____ Discuss discharge follow-up with patient.

Evaluative Criteria:

_____ Students who have created the scenario use the nursing process to cue the observing students to make recommendations about patient care. Cues are adequate for recognition by the observing students.

_____ Students observing were able to recognize signs and symptoms as wound infection and pulmonary embolism.

_____ Students observing were able to recommend scenario students follow diagnostic protocol to assess and begin interventions for wound infection and pulmonary embolism.

_____ Students observing were able to connect the immobility related to a wound infection with the consequence of pulmonary embolism.

_____ Student observing were able to accurately assess abnormal lab test and diagnostic test and suggest treatment.

_____ Students observing were able to suggest correct medication and dosages to treat patient's condition.

_____ Patient stabilizes for discharge, and students recommend proper home care follow-up.

_____ Students observing and participating recognize communication issues and discuss how effective communication and teamwork would improve outcomes in this scenario.

G. Debriefing Guidelines

Instructors worked with the student scenario creators to create objectives and outcomes for each scenario. General questions reviewed in the debriefing were as follows:

1. What disease process was being portrayed in the scenario?
2. What were the key assessment factors and vital sign parameters important in the scenario?
3. Did the scenario follow the known standard of care for the medical-surgical problem?
4. Was there anything new that you learned as a result of the scenario?
5. What were the crucial nursing interventions and evaluation points necessary for the patient's condition to improve?
6. Was the scenario realistic and engaging?

H. Suggestions/Key Features to Replicate or Improve

These student generated scenarios are an excellent synthesis exercise in which students are required to access all knowledge and skills learned in order to evaluate their peers with regard to their knowledge and skills. Posting the assignment gave students time to review and ask questions of their individual instructors. In addition, the use and access to the entire lab and all equipment was important to promote the "realness" of the simulation. Students were encouraged to be as creative as possible throughout the scenario generation, which seemed to be a very enjoyable part of the exercise. Students showed enthusiasm for all roles, including running the computer program, which we believed might have been a hindrance. The students demonstrated how quickly they are able to learn and adapt to new technology as active participants in a nonthreatening and collaborative setting.

I. Recommendations for Further Use

Student-generated scenarios should be utilized as a creative and exciting alternative to testing. We have all found that even in the best faculty-developed scenarios, students have ideas and suggestions that change the running of scenarios written by instructors. This format, although not appropriate at the lower levels, allows students to show what they know in a safe, supportive environment while testing knowledge, skills, and critical thinking of the graduating senior. The instructor role became one of support, encouragement, and resource person. At least one instructor was recruited into the scenario to play a role. Instructors commented they were "amazed" at how well the students did and how comprehensive the student-generated scenarios were.

J. Discussion of Simulation-Based Pedagogy and How This New Technology Has Contributed to Improved Student Outcomes

Simulation-based pedagogy has contributed to improved student outcomes in two significant ways: improved demonstration of critical thinking abilities, and knowledge-based application of principles of safety, communication, and team collaboration.

In student-generated scenarios, each group of students found that there was a need to outline the case being presented from a critical-thinking perspective. Each scenario needed to be complete and accurate but also to be able to anticipate the critical thinking of the other students through cueing the students observing to help them move along in the scenario. Once all the pertinent facts of the case were checked and verified, the chart was set up and the students had to ask, "Will they recognize this as abnormal and know what to do?" Using their own knowledge and checking references available, the students then were able to piece together the scenario using the nursing process as a template for how the other students would process information and come to conclusions. Senior students found that the use of the nursing process facilitated the learning of the other students during the scenario and in debriefing.

Safety, communication and team collaboration were essential in the successful development and implementation of the scenario. Safety issues were addressed repeatedly without guidance of the instructors and in fact were often used as a part of the scenario in need of recognition and correction during the scenarios. Communication between nurses, patients, families, and other health care providers was also an essential element of each scenario. Effective communication resulted in improved patient outcomes during the simulations. Teamwork and collaboration with members of the health care team were emphasized in each simulation. As the simulations evolved, the observing students made recommendations, and each team member worked together to carry out nursing interventions. Included as part of the team were family members, used in order to clarify and explain the circumstances surrounding the scenario.

Students commented that this type of scenario made them realize how much more they knew than previously thought. Most students commented how much more confident they felt in their abilities after doing these simulations. In addition, students suggested that more simulation within the curriculum would be beneficial at all levels of the program.

In summary, we thought student-generated scenarios contributed not only to increased application of critical thinking, safety, communication, and teamwork but also to increased levels of confidence of graduating seniors. In this way, student-generated scenarios, as an end point learning exercise for graduating seniors, affirms the use of simulation-based pedagogy not only as a test of competency but as a demonstration of the skill and knowledge level required at the end of an undergraduate nursing program.

References

Larew, C., Lessans, S., Spunt, D., Foster, D., & Covington, B. G. (2006). Application of Benner's theory in an interactive simulation. *Nursing Education Perspectives, 27*(1), 16–21.

Laerdal Medical. (2008a). *Scenario planning worksheet.* Retrieved May10th 2008, from http://simulation.laerdal.com/forum/files/folders/checklists_worksheets/entry8.aspx

Laerdal Medical. (2008b). *Scenario validation checklist.* Retrieved May 10, 2008, from http://simulation.laerdal.com/forum/files/folders/checklists_worksheets/entry9.aspx

National Council of State Boards of Nursing. (2007). *NCLEX-RN examination: Test plan for the National Council Licensure Examination for Registered Nurses.* Retrieved June 18, 2008, from https://www.ncsbn.org/RN_Test_Plan_2007_Web.pdf

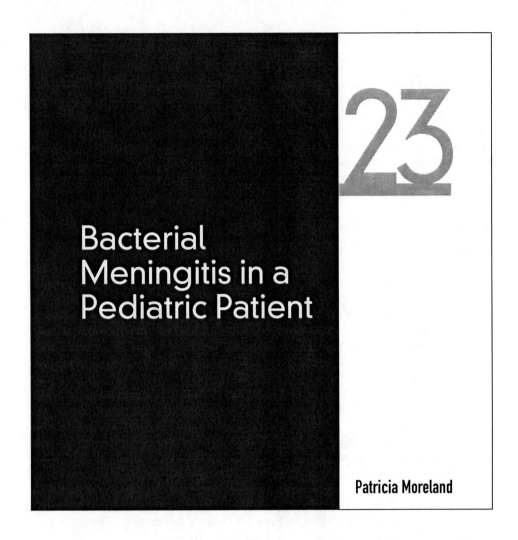

23

Bacterial Meningitis in a Pediatric Patient

Patricia Moreland

A. Discussion of Implementation of Simulation-Based Pedagogy in Each Contributor's Individualized Teaching

There is widespread recognition that caring for children and their families requires a unique set of knowledge and skills (Lambton, 2008). The anatomy and physiology of a child differs markedly from that of an adult. These fundamental differences and developmental factors affect how a child responds to illness and injury. In addition, the pattern of disease and presentation of symptoms often varies with the age of the child. Knowledge of disease processes and the ability to recognize subtle signs of deterioration in a child are imperative to provide safe and effective care. Moreover, understanding the complex needs of families of ill children requires sensitivity and good communication skills (Ryan & Steinmiller, 2004).

Educators face the challenge of providing students with optimal opportunities to learn the critical thinking skills necessary to care for children. However, current resources for pediatric clinical experience are becoming less available. The limited number of clinical facilities, lack of breadth of clinical experiences, and current shortage of nursing faculty has resulted in barriers to acquisition of

clinical skills. Time constraints as well as safety factors also limit a student's opportunity to apply problem-solving methods in the pediatric setting. Simulation
technology allows students to duplicate the types of scenarios that they are likely
to encounter in clinical practice. Further, simulation provides the student an opportunity to perform procedures in a safe environment and to receive immediate
feedback. Students can develop effective communication skills and discuss issues that concern them prior to being confronted with issues in the real world.

B. Description of Educational Materials Available in Your Teaching Area and Relative to Your Specialty

Western Connecticut State University has had a dedicated pediatric simulation laboratory since 2007. The pediatric laboratory is designed to approximate
an in-patient hospital room. The pediatric human patient simulator (HPS),
VitalSim®, is the intermediate-fidelity mannequin used in the pediatric laboratory. VitalSim® is the size of a 6-year-old male HPS that simulates "real"
responses to critical injury and medical interventions. He features realistic pulmonary, cardiovascular, and gastrointestinal systems and can be programmed
to display normal and abnormal findings. These physiologic responses provide
nursing students with realistic responses to their nursing interventions and increase their critical-thinking skills. Presently, VitalSim® is used to demonstrate
and practice pediatric physical assessment, disease-based scenarios, growth
and development assessment, and pharmacologic interventions. Pediatric skills
practiced include intramuscular injections and urinary catherization. Additional
educational materials available in the pediatric simulation laboratory include a
pediatric medication cart, emergency equipment (ambu bag, oxygen, endotracheal tubes, intraosseous catheter), Broslow tape, IV equipment, feeding tubes,
cardiac electrodes, pulse oximeter, and suction equipment.

C. Specific Objective for Simulation Utilization Within a Specific Course and the Overall Program

The primary objective for this scenario is to assess the student's ability to conduct a thorough pediatric neurologic assessment, recognize abnormal neurologic findings, and develop a plan of care for a pediatric patient with bacterial
meningitis. This scenario was designed for third- and fourth-year BSN students
or first-year ADN students. The scenario would take place during the third week
of clinical, following a lecture on pediatric physical exam, meningitis, communication skills, and health history. Students will have attended two clinical experiences and demonstrated a pediatric physical exam under the supervision of a
clinical instructor. Because self-assessment is so important to the development
of a reflective practitioner, several tools were examined and adapted to address
the needs of the assessment of pediatric patients (Ball & Bindler, 2008; LaRock,
2008). The self-assessment form shown in Table 23.1 was developed to meet
the needs of this scenario. Students are required to fill out the form prior to the
simulation and then are evaluated during debriefing.

23.1 Physical Examination of a Pediatric Patient Student Self-Assessment

NAME _____ DATE _____

Directions: The following statements ask how confident you feel about your ability to conduct a pediatric physical exam. Please check the box corresponding to the number that best describes your level of confidence doing each activity. Assume that you have to do each activity during your NEXT CLINICAL DAY.

1 = not at all confident, 2 = somewhat confident, 3 = very confident

General	1	2	3
Assess general appearance, nutrition status			
Assess speech and language abilities appropriate for child's age			
Assess body posture, symmetry of movement			

Vital Signs	1	2	3
Assess blood pressure			
Assess apical and radial pulse			
Assess respiratory rate			
Pulse oximeter			
Note normal findings for child's age			
Identify normal variations in vital signs related to pain, anxiety, fever			

Skin	1	2	3
Assess texture, temperature, mobility, turgor, tenderness, moisture, and color throughout exam			
Note ecchymosis, rashes, petechiae, purpura			

Head/Face	1	2	3
Inspect shape and symmetry of head			
Inspect face for dysmorphic features, symmetry of facial muscles			
Observe head lag in infant			
Palpate skull for evidence of trauma			
Palpate anterior and posterior fontanel			
Assess CN V, CN VII			
Measure head circumference (until age 3 years)			

Eyes	1	2	3
Inspect conjunctiva and sclera			
Pupillary reaction			
Identify ptosis & strabismus			

(continued)

Ears	1	2	3
Assess placement			
Observe for rhinorrhea			
Palpate mastoid process			
Nose & Sinuses	1	2	3
Inspect nasal mucosa			
Palpate sinuses for tenderness			
Observe for nasal flaring			
Observe for rhinorrhea			
Mouth & Pharynx	1	2	3
Inspect lips and buccal mucosa for color, symmetry, moisture, sores			
Inspect tonsils and oropharynx			
Neck	1	2	3
Palpate lymph nodes			
Assess range of motion			
Chest & Lungs	1	2	3
Inspect shape and contour of thorax			
Assess for retractions (intercostals, substernal, suprasternal)			
Auscultate for wheezes, ronchi, or stridor			
Heart & Peripheral Perfusion	1	2	3
Ausculate heart sounds aortic, pulmonic, tricuspid, mitral areas			
Identify "normal range" heart rate for infant/child			
Auscultate for murmurs			
Palpate peripheral pulses (brachial, radial, femoral, pedal)			
Extremity warmth			
Capillary refill			
Abdomen	1	2	3
Inspect abdomen for size and shape			
Inspect umbilicus in a newborn			
Auscultate for bowel sounds			
Palpate for liver size			
Palpate spleen			
Palpate for tenderness, firmness, or masses			
Genitalia & Anus	1	2	3
Female: Observe labia majora, labia minora			
Male: Urinary meatus, testes, circumcision			

(continued)

Musculoskeletal System	1	2	3
Range of motion			
Muscle strength/tone			
Redness, tenderness of joints			
Neurologic System	1	2	3
Level of consciousness			
Observe spontaneous activity for symmetry and smoothness of movement			
Assess balance and coordination (standing/walking)			
Assess sensory function			
Assess deep tendon reflexes			
Assess rooting reflex of an infant			
Assess sucking reflex of an infant			
Assess acoustic blink reflex of an infant			
Assess palmar & plantar grasp at birth			
Assess stepping in infant to 8 weeks of age			

Student Learning Activities

1. Review and practice pediatric assessment.
2. Review pathophysiology, assessment, and treatment of meningitis.
3. Review good communication techniques.
4. Review calculations of safe dosage of medications and IV fluids.

D. Introduction of Scenario to Include Setting the Scene, Technology Used, Objectives, and Description of Participants

Setting the Scene:

Equipment needed: Pediatric ambu bag/mask, oxygen mask, suction equipment, patient name bracelet, allergy bracelet with "Keflex" written in red, pulse oximeter, stethoscopes (alcohol swabs), BP cuff, intravenous setup with Burretrol (0.9 normal saline), Oucher scale, thermometer, Cefotaxime vials, Tylenol (liquid), Decadron vial, syringes, needles, medicine cups
Red rash (petechia) placed on chest and upper extremities.

Resources needed: Pediatric textbook, pediatric drug book, computer access for database search

Simulator level: VitalSim®, an intermediate-fidelity HPS

Participants needed: Students to act as parent, physician, and recorder of scenario, and student to calculate drug dosages and IV rates. The remainder of the students (4) will decide as a group on the care of the child and the family. Faculty member will provide patient information and adjust settings on VitalSim®.

Objectives

1. Student will use the nursing process to demonstrate the proper management of a child with bacterial meningitis.
2. Student will provide interventions within the scenario that maintains a standard of care, therapeutic communication, safety precautions, and psychosocial care.

The National Council of State Boards of Nursing's *National Council Licensure Examination for Registered Nurses* (NCLEX-RN) test plan categories and subcategories (NCSBN, 2007) addressed in the simulation are as follows:

> Safe and Effective Care Environment
> > *Management of Care*
> > > Establishing Priorities
> > > Legal Rights and Responsibilities
> > *Safety and Infection Control*
> > > Standard/Transmission-Based/Other Precautions
> > > Safe Use of Equipment
> Health Promotion and Maintenance
> > Techniques of Physical Assessment
> > *Psychosocial Integrity*
> > > Coping Mechanisms
> > > Therapeutic Communications
> Physiological Integrity
> > *Basic Care and Comfort*
> > > Elimination
> > > Non-Pharmacological Comfort Interventions
> > *Pharmacological and Parenteral Therapies*
> > > Dosage Calculation
> > > Medication Administration
> > > Parenteral/Intravenous Therapies
> > > Pharmacological Agents/Actions
> > > Pharmacological Pain Management
> > *Reduction of Risk Potential*
> > > Laboratory Values
> > > Diagnostic Tests
> > > Vital Signs
> > *Physiological Adaptation*
> > > Hemodynamics
> > > Illness Management

E. Describe Running of the Scenario

The scenario will begin in the Emergency Department (ED) of a very busy pediatric hospital. At the time of the child's arrival, the ED is caring for four trauma patients from a motor vehicle accident. The mother of the child appears anxious as she walks into what appears to be a very chaotic, noisy environment.

Role-play: Description for Anthony's mother
You are the mother of Anthony, a 4-year-old boy. You have brought him to the ED because he has a high fever and has been vomiting. You have been up all night with Anthony and you are very tired and moderately anxious about your son's condition. You expect the nurse caring for Anthony to be able to answer all of your questions. During the course of the scenario, you will ask the following questions in any order:

"What is happening to my son?"
"Why is he having those 'staring episodes'?"
"Could this illness have been prevented?"
"Anthony is hungry. Can he have the McDonald's hamburger I brought for him?"
"Why are you giving him Tylenol?"
"Why are you putting Anthony on the cardiac monitor? He doesn't have any heart problems."
"What can I do to help him?"
"I want to stay with Anthony when he has his lumbar puncture. I am not going to leave him!"

F. Presentation of Completed Template

Title: Bacterial Meningitis
Nursing 325

Focus Area:
Pediatrics

Scenario Description:
The students arrive in the ED of a large tertiary pediatric hospital. They are assigned to care for a 4-year-old male who has just arrived per ambulance. Report is given to student by the Emergency Medical Staff (EMS) and the day-shift nurse.

> *History of present illness:* Anthony is a 4-year-old black male with a history of fever and decreased activity of 1 day duration. Anthony's temperature during the night was 104, for which he received Tylenol at 0200. Anthony has vomited twice this am and now refuses all liquids. Mother states that child has had several "staring episodes" this am. His past medical history is unremarkable except for diagnosis of bilateral otitis media 1 week prior to admission. Pediatrician ordered amoxicillin for otitis; however, mother was unable to fill prescription due to lack of health insurance. Anthony lives with his parents, a 2-year-old sister, and a 12-month-old brother. He attends day care 3 days a week while his mother works at a local school.
>
> On entering the room, students find a pale, 4-year-old male lying quietly in a dark room. Child does not open his eyes but answers questions appropriately. Speech is slow and deliberate. Anthony is irritable and grimaces with any movement. He is reluctant to lift his head and complains of an occipital headache. Mother is at bedside.

Weight: 38 lb
Allergies: Keflex
Past medical history: As above
Medications: None
Immunizations: Up to date
Developmental history: Normal
Family History: Unremarkable except 2-year-old sister has history of febrile seizures
Social history: Family just moved to area and does not have family or friends living near by

Scenario Implementation:
Initial Settings for Human Patient Simulator

HR: 120, RR: 48, BP 93/50
Pulse oximeter: 98%
Place cloth over child's forehead.
Place ambu bag/mask, oxygen mask, suction catheter in room near bed.

Objectives

1. Demonstrates effective communication (e.g., listening, advising, counseling) with family and the interdisciplinary health care team.
2. Performs a thorough clinical assessment of a pediatric patient.
3. Recognizes risk factors related to meningitis.
4. Recognizes the signs and symptoms of meningitis.
5. Initiate therapy for a child with increased intracranial pressure.
6. Initiates proper safety precautions related to increased ICP (seizures).
7. Recognition of abnormal lab findings (CBC, electrolytes, CSF).
8. Evaluate effectiveness of therapeutic interventions.
9. Identifies social issues related to access to health care.

Required Student Assessments and Actions

_____ Introduce self to child and family.
_____ Identify patient by name band.
_____ Perform a rapid evaluation of child's general condition, including airway, respiratory status and cardiovascular status.
_____ Apply cardiac monitor.
_____ Apply pulse oximeter.
_____ Assess child's level of consciousness (asks questions appropriate for 4 year old, knows teacher's name and sibling names, identifies mother, states favorite cartoon or game)
_____ Assess pupillary reaction.
_____ Perform a focused neurologic examination (muscle strength, muscle tone, deep tendon reflexes).
_____ Perform examination to assess Kernig sign.
_____ Perform examination to assess Brudzinski sign.

_____ Assess hydration status (mucous membranes, skin turgor, urine output).
_____ Assess skin for rash (petechia).
_____ Ask parent about his or her impression of child's condition.
_____ Elevate head of bed 15 to 30 degrees to decrease ICP.
_____ Assess child's level of pain (uses Oucher scale and finds pain level 7).
_____ Administer Tylenol for headache.
_____ Recognize that allergy to Keflex is contraindication to administer cefo-taxime.
_____ Administer ampicillin following lumbar puncture.
_____ Administer IV fluid rate based on child's weight.
_____ Re-evaluate level pain.
_____ Find pain level decreased to 3.
_____ Re-evaluate level of consciousness.
_____ Find child alert and orientated.
_____ Evaluate lab values and communicates with physician (CBC, electrolytes, CSF).

Instructor Interventions

- Direct students' care of child.
- Answer questions.
- Check medication and IV fluid calculations according to guidelines (shown below).

Medication Calculations

Weight: Convert 38 lb to kilograms = $38 \div 2.2 = 17$ kg

Tylenol elixir: Dose ordered—15 mg per kg q 4 hours prn temp >100.4
15 mg $\times 17$ kg $= 255$ mg per dose
Tylenol supplied 160 mg/5 mL
255 mg $= 8$ mL
Ampicillin: Dose ordered—200 mg/kg/24 hours q 4 hours
200 mg $\times 17$ kg $= 3,400$ mg in 24 hours
$3,400$ mg $\div 6 = 566$ mg per dose
Dexamethasone: Dose ordered—0.15 mg/kg/dose q 6 hours
0.15 mg $\times 17$ kg $= 2.5$ mg

IV Fluid Calculations

IV fluids: D5 .45 normal saline
Calculation for hourly maintenance rate for pediatric patients:
Up to 10 kg = 100 mL/kg $\div$ 24 hours
11–20 kg = 1,000 + 50 mL/kg for each kg above 10 kg $\div$ 24 hours
Above 20 kg = 1,500 + 20 mL/kg for each kg above 20 kg $\div$ 24 hours

A.L. hourly maintenance fluid rate:
Weight 17 kg = 1,000 + 50 mL/kg for each kg above 10 kg $\div$ 24 hours
$1,000 + 50 \times 7(17$ kg $- 10$ kg$) = 1,000 + 350 = 1,350 \div$ 24 hours $= 1350 \div 24$ hours $= 56$ mL/hour

Evaluation Criteria:

_____ Student identifies self and patient properly.
_____ Apply cardiac monitor.
_____ Apply pulse oximeter.
_____ Assess child's level of consciousness.
_____ Perform neurologic assessment.
_____ Identify risk factors for meningitis.
_____ Demonstrate Kernig sign.
_____ Demonstrate Brudzinski sign.
_____ Identify rash as petechia.
_____ Elevate head of bed 15 to 30 degrees.
_____ Use Oucher scale to assess pain.
_____ Calculate correct dose of Tylenol.
_____ Calculate correct IV rate.
_____ Evaluate CSF results.

G. Debriefing Guidelines

1. Was it difficult to do a physical exam on the child with the parent present?
2. Did the nurse communicate at the developmental level of the child?
3. Did the nurse communicate effectively with the parent about the nursing interventions to be implemented?
4. Did the nurse act as an advocate for the child regarding pain control?
5. Did the nurse act as an advocate for the family to facilitate family presence during an invasive procedure?
6. Identify three nursing diagnoses related to your physical exam.
7. Were safety precautions taken at all times?
8. What psychosocial issues needed to be addressed?
9. What was done well?
10. What could be improved?

H. Suggestions/Key Features to Replicate or Improve

This scenario has not been fully implemented into the pediatric curriculum. A case study version of the scenario has been used previously without simulation technology. To replicate this scenario, students could be provided a research article on the current management of meningitis to assist with their preparation. The realism of the scenario could be enhanced by including both the mother and the father and incorporating a script for each. Emphasis on communication skills with child, parents, and other health care personnel would be beneficial.

I. Recommendations for Further Use

Integrating simulation technology into pediatric seminar enhances the student's learning process. The use of HPS allows students to evaluate their knowledge and skills in a "real-life" situation. This scenario can be altered to present the concepts of septic shock, seizures, and DIC.

J. Discussion of Simulation-Based Pedagogy and How This New Technology Has Contributed to Improved Student Outcomes

Research supports that students in pediatric courses experience a significant amount of stress while caring for patients (Oermann & Lukomski, 2001). Fear of making errors and difficulties with interactions between the student and family members have been identified as stressors. Understanding the need for extensive knowledge and specialized skills to care for a pediatric patient requires the development of creative learning opportunities. Simulation-based knowledge can provide the opportunity for students to develop assessment skills, understand unique pediatric diseases, and develop competencies for nursing care. Students can practice effective communication techniques and learn to interact with families in a crisis situation within a safe environment.

References

Ball, J., & Bindler, R. (2008). Pediatric assessment. In *Pediatric nursing: Caring for children* (4th ed., pp. 149–210). Upper Saddle River, NJ: Pearson Prentice Hall.

Lambton, J. (2008). Integrating simulation into a pediatric nursing curriculum: A 25% solution? *Simulation in Healthcare, 3*, 53–57.

LaRock, W. (2008). *Evaluation of a nurse mentor training program in Eastern Cape, South Africa.* Unpublished doctoral dissertation, Columbia University.

National Council of State Boards of Nursing. (2007). *NCLEX-RN examination: Test plan for the National Council Licensure Examination for Registered Nurses.* Retrieved June 18, 2008, from https://www.ncsbn.org/RN_Test_Plan_2007_Web.pdf

Oermann, M., & Lukomski, A. (2001). Experiences of students in pediatric nursing clinical courses. *Journal for Specialists in Pediatric Nursing, 6*(2), 65–72.

Ryan, E., & Steinmiller, E. (2004). Modeling family-centered pediatric nursing care: Strategies for shift report. *Journal for Specialists in Pediatric Nursing, 9*(4), 123–134.

Recommended Readings

Fiedor, M. (2004). Pediatric simulation: A valuable tool for pediatric medical education. *Critical Care Medicine, 32*(2), S72–S74.

Prober, C. (2007). Central nervous systems infections. In R. Kliegman, R. Behrman, H. Jenson, & B. Stanton (Eds.), *Nelson's textbook of pediatrics* (18th ed., pp. 2512–2521). Philadelphia: Saunders Elsevier.

Robertson, J., & Shilkofski, N. (2005). Drug formulary. In *The Harriet Lane handbook* (17th ed., pp. 697–1003). Philadelphia: Elsevier Mosby.

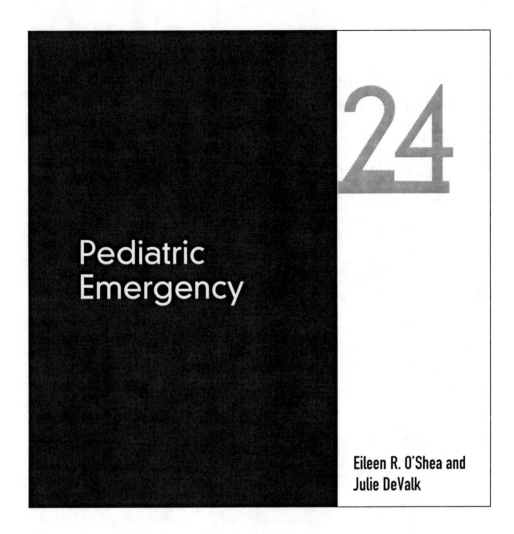

24

Pediatric Emergency

Eileen R. O'Shea and
Julie DeValk

This chapter will focus on the critical thought process and interaction among the entire medical team when encountering an inpatient pediatric emergency. The following scenario was trialed several times on two different acute-care pediatric medical-surgical units. The goal of the scenario was to better prepare the new and experienced bedside nurse by building confidence and decreasing anxiety during emergency situations. As suggested in the literature, the bedside nurse is most often the first responder and first link in the chain of survival for a patient in distress (Hunt, Walker, Shaffner, Miller, & Pronovost, 2008). Hence, it is critical for nurses to be proficient in their role as effective communicators and coordinators of care during an emergency.

Although this simulation was designed for actual staff nurses, it can be adapted easily for the undergraduate nursing student. Schools of nursing have recognized that preparing new nurses for emergency situations is essential, and simulations can help to bridge both the theoretical with the clinical components of this learning (Spunt, Foster, & Adams, 2004).

A. Discussion of Implementation of Simulation-Based Pedagogy in Each Contributor's Individualized Teaching

This project began with an experienced staff nurse (clinical nurse II) recognizing the need for confidence and enhanced skills among staff nurses in emergency situations on a general pediatric unit. With each emergency situation, it was not uncommon to observe a state of commotion among the staff. Many times, the bedside nurse would not remain with his or her patient, in order to search for equipment or to summon physicians. As a result, the bedside nurse was often not present to provide a clear patient history when the emergency medical response team arrived.

In contrast, the medical doctors (MDs) participated in mock scenarios on a routine basis to help interns gain confidence and knowledge when confronted with an actual emergency. With this concept in mind, nursing approached the unit hospitalist and chief physicians to develop a more collaborative and interdisciplinary model, which would include the bedside nurse. The MDs were eager and willing for this project to get under way. To prepare the unit nurses for the upcoming simulations, a survey was developed. The survey served two purposes. First, it was used to gather information regarding nurses' level of confidence in emergency situations. Second, the survey asked if the staff would find this experience beneficial for their work. Results showed that more than 90% of nurses strongly agreed that they lacked confidence in emergency situations and would benefit from the program as described in the survey.

To improve communication among all participants involved in the emergency scenario, the staff agreed to utilize the SBAR technique, which stands for *situation, background, assessment,* and *recommendation* (The SBAR Technique, 2005). This strategy provides a standardized approach for individuals to effectively communicate and is currently being used by health care providers nationwide. The SBAR technique is also being trialed within several student nurse clinical experiences. The method serves as a framework for the nursing students when delivering "hand-off" communication to their instructors and preceptors (SBAR for Students, 2007).

B. Description of Educational Materials Available in Your Teaching Area and Relative to Your Specialty

This scenario took place at a major university-affiliated children's hospital in the Northeast. The treatment room on an inpatient pediatric unit was the designated site for the simulation. The room is fully equipped with the following:

- Stretcher
- Full cardiac/apnea monitor
- Suction headwall unit
- Oxygen with flow meter (high and low flow meter)
- IV pump and pole
- EKG machine
- Static manikin

- Fully stocked code cart with defibrillator
- Backboard
- Sharps container
- Gloves
- Blood pressure cuff (neonate and child size)
- Bag valve mask and various masks
- IV and blood supplies
- Cabinets with various child life props

C. Specific Objective for Simulation Utilization Within a Specific Course and the Overall Program

The primary objective of this scenario was for the bedside staff nurse to recognize a pediatric emergency and to utilize a collaborative approach in problem solving with the goal of stabilizing the patient. This scenario is designed to assist both the novice and experienced nurse. It takes approximately 20 minutes to implement the scenario and an additional 20 minutes to debrief afterward. It is the goal for this program to be conducted on a bimonthly basis. Currently, the individuals are selected at random to participate at the mutual convenience of both the medical and nursing staff.

Specific Course Objectives Met With This Scenario

1. Synthesizes knowledge from the arts, sciences, and nursing in the provision of holistic care for children and their families experiencing alterations in health/development.
2. Employs critical-thinking skills in analyzing and responding to complex clinical situations.
3. Uses creative and developmentally appropriate communication strategies with children.
4. Demonstrates accountability and fiscal responsibility in nursing care of children and families.
5. Collaborates with children, their families, and other health care providers in the planning, delivery, and evaluation of holistic care.
6. Provides and promotes evidence-based, culturally sensitive, and ethically sound nursing care.
7. Demonstrates professional accountability and responsibility in performing all aspects of the nursing student role.

Undergraduate Program Objectives

1. Demonstrate effectiveness in planning and providing therapeutic nursing care, managing information, and promoting self-care competence of culturally diverse individuals, families, groups, and communities.
2. Employ a variety of technologies and other therapeutic modalities with sensitivity for the provision of care.
3. Make sound clinical judgments based on nursing science and related theory, using critical thinking, and ethical decision making.

4. Demonstrate collaboration with peers, patient, health care professionals, and others within health care teams in the process of planning, delegating, implementing, and evaluating care.
5. Communicate with clarity, purpose, and sensitivity using a variety of methods, including technology.
6. Advocate for patients, consumers, and the nursing profession through involvement in the political process and health/patient care policies and practices.

D. Introduction of Scenario to Include Setting the Scene, Technology Used, Objectives, and Description of Participants

Setting the Scene and Technology Used

A 14-year-old bicyclist with no helmet was hit by a car. He was seen in the Emergency Department (ED), where he was evaluated and deemed stable. A CT scan of the head was determined to be negative. The patient was admitted to the general floor for observation overnight. Two hours after arriving on the unit, the patient called out to the nurse complaining of severe abdominal pain.

Objectives

1. The student will utilize critical-thinking skills to assess an acute change in presentation of abdominal pain.
2. The student will perform a focused abdominal exam and pain assessment, including vital signs.
3. The student will collaborate with an interprofessional health care team during an emergency situation.
4. The student will communicate to the emergency response team using the SBAR format (situation, background, assessment, and recommendation).
5. The student will delegate appropriately to ancillary health care workers.
6. The student will use developmentally appropriate communication with the patient.

The National Council of State Boards of Nursing's National Council Licensure Examination for Registered Nurses (NCLEX-RN) test plan categories and subcategories (NCSBN, 2007) addressed in the simulation are as follows:

    Safe and Effective Care Environment
        Management of Care
            Collaboration With Interdisciplinary Team (physician, RN, PCA)
            Delegation
            Establishing Priorities
        Safety and Infection Control
            Safe Use of Equipment
            Standard/Transmission-Based/Other Precautions (IV start)

Health Promotion and Maintenance
     Developmental Stages (teen) and Transitions
     Techniques of Physical Assessment
Psychosocial Integrity
     Therapeutic Communications
Physiological Integrity
     Pharmacological and Parenteral Therapies
     Parenteral/Intravenous Therapies
     Reduction of Risk Potential
     Laboratory Values
     Vitals Signs
     Physiological Adaptation
     Hemodynamics
     Medical Emergencies

Description of Participants

This emergency scenario will need five participants and one manikin to be effective.

1. *Teen:* The static manikin was used for this scenario. However, utilizing a medium- or high-fidelity human patient simulator (HPS) would enhance the reality of this simulation by allowing for changing vitals signs and physical exam. The manikin should be dressed in a hospital gown with a wristband containing the patient name and medical record number.
2. *Bedside RN/Student RN:* The student nurse should have had a health assessment course, basic fundamental skills course, and medical-surgical and pediatric nursing courses in which content related to an acute abdomen and interventions would have been previously learned. The learner should be confident in the following skills: connecting a patient to a cardiac/respiratory monitor; providing a focused abdominal and pain assessment; obtaining frequent vital signs and monitoring oxygen saturations; hanging IV fluids; and connecting a bag valve mask to oxygen. Knowing the roles of health care team members during a code is necessary as well as communicating to the team using the SBAR format (situation, background, assessment, and recommendation).
3. *RN/Patient care assistant "runner":* The runner should be an additional student or volunteer whose role is to be a support person for the bedside nurse. He or she may have to leave the room to make phone calls or to retrieve equipment and supplies.
4. *RN recorder:* This will be another student/volunteer person whose job will be to record the order of events and interventions. He or she should not leave the room to help the runner.
5. *MD/Resident:* This volunteer will ask the bedside nurse for a history of the patient and will be providing verbal orders throughout the scenario.
6. *Faculty instructor/Handler:* The instructor should be present to assist participants through the progression of the scenario. He or she should describe the patient's current mental status and initial vital signs and reinforce the major complaint of abdominal pain. Additionally, the instructor will be responsible

for describing changes in the teen's abdomen, which progresses to a rigid state, with deteriorating vital signs. These changes can be indicated by using index cards. The final index card should show a low blood pressure, decreasing oxygenation, and the patient experiencing a loss of consciousness. The instructor should also take notes during the simulation so that they can be utilized during the debriefing.

E. Describe Running of the Scenario

Prior to the scenario, the treatment room was prepared with child static manikin dressed in a gown. The unit hospitalist, the chief MD, and RN in charge of the project were all present as "handlers," not actual participants. Once the bedside RN entered the room, the chief MD (handler) provided some background information, including the patient's current mental status and initial vital signs and reinforced the major complaint of abdominal pain. The scenario progressed over the course of 20 minutes with the patient steadily decompensating.

F. Presentation of Completed Template

Didactic Preparation

In preparation for this scenario, the student will need to have read content related to pediatric abdominal injury, pediatric vital sign norms for a teen, SBAR communication technique (The SBAR Technique, 2005), and the role of nursing during emergency codes. Additionally, the learner should be prepared to engage in communication with the teen. The psychomotor skills to be performed include focused abdominal and pain assessment, vital signs, and preparation and maintenance of IV fluids.

Assessment Tools

To assess the teen's pain, a self-report numeric scale can be utilized.

Title: Pediatric Emergency

Focus Area:
Pediatric Nursing or Critical Care Nursing

Scenario Description:
The chief MD and RN in charge of the project coordinated the time and place for the scenario. A nurse was selected at random and summoned to the treatment room for an emergency. It was prearranged with the charge nurse on the unit that she would cover the RN's assignment while she was participating in the scenario. On entering the treatment room, the nurse discovered there was a 14-year-old boy on a stretcher.

> *Patient:* Pediatric patient
> *Age:* 14 years

History: Normal healthy child until earlier in evening, when he was struck by a motor vehicle while riding a bicycle without a helmet.

Handler script: "The 14-year-old boy was lying in bed with a chief complaint of abdominal pain in the left upper quadrant. Less than 12 hours prior, he had been seen in the ED after being struck by a motor vehicle while riding his bicycle without a helmet. A head CT was performed and was negative. The patient was deemed stable and sent to the inpatient general unit for observation. His vital signs were initially stable; he had no IV access and had not previously required any pain medication."

Scenario Objectives:

1. The student will utilize critical-thinking skills to assess an acute change in presentation of abdominal pain.
2. The student will perform a focused abdominal exam and pain assessment, including vital signs.
3. The student will collaborate with an interprofessional health care team during an emergency situation.
4. The student will communicate to the emergency response team using the SBAR format (situation, background, assessment, and recommendation).
5. The student will delegate appropriately to ancillary health care workers.
6. The student will use developmentally appropriate communication with the patient.

Setting the Scene:

Equipment needed:

- Static manikin (child/teen)
- Monitor with heart rate and pulse oximeter capabilities
- Monitor leads/oximeter sensor
- BP cuff and stethoscope
- IV pump and blood drawing/IV insertion supplies
- Gloves
- Suction setup
- Bag valve mask, oxygen setup with high flow meter

Resources needed:
- Emergency recorder list

Participant roles:
- Handler to field questions from RN and intern/resident as well as progressing verbally through scenario with patient's deteriorating condition
- Bedside RN to perform assessment and effectively relay information to arriving MDs to bedside
- RN/Patient care assistant delegated to "run" for equipment and supplies

- RN to record emergency
- MD to identify who is main physician in charge and request various orders to be carried out by bedside nurse

Scenario Implementation:

Initial Settings

- Brief history of patient condition and chief complaint presented by handler/instructor
- Information regarding tests already performed in ED and results
- Presented with initial vital signs via index cards held by handler (or set on a high-fidelity HPS)
- IV supplies available

Required Assessments and Actions

- Introduce self and role.
- Place patient on monitor and obtain set of vital signs.
- Auscultate abdomen and perform abdominal and pain assessment.
- Ask handler if any pain meds on board.
- Page intern to bedside for assistance when BP noted to be dropping.
- Give clear history of patient condition to arriving MD, using the SBAR format.
- Follow through with orders from MD in charge to place IV and start IV fluids.
- Delegate to other nurses to run for supplies and equipment.
- Summon other nurses to bedside to assist with IV placement and commencing of IV fluids.
- Delegate to another nurse/PCA to page pediatric surgery stat.
- Has code cart standing by.
- Continue with frequent vital signs.
- Delegate to another nurse/PCA to page respiratory therapist.
- Assist MD with maintaining airway once oxygen saturations too low and needing ventilation until respiratory therapist arrives and takes over.
- Ensure someone is recording events.
- Prepare patient for immediate transfer to operating room.

Handler Interventions

- Progressing through scenario, describe changes in VS, rigid abdomen
- Subsequent deteriorating vital signs held up periodically through scenario by handler (or changing with programming of minimum or high-fidelity HPS)
- Simulation of patient's deteriorating status and subsequent crashing BP and loss of consciousness
- Debriefing

Evaluation Criteria:

Checklist of Interventions and Assessments

_____ Introduce self.
_____ Put patient on monitor.
_____ Perform focused abdominal assessment.
_____ Perform pain assessment on a scale of 1 to 10.
_____ Note patient has had no pain med on board.
_____ Note patient's initial and worsening vital signs.
_____ Note patient has no IV access.
_____ Suggest IV access and fluids and places IV.
_____ Stay at bedside at all times and delegates to others for supplies.
_____ Summon intern to bedside.
_____ Give clear patient history to MDs arriving at bedside using the SBAR format.
_____ Clearly establish who is "in charge" and takes orders only from that person.
_____ Call Code when patient is deteriorating and needing extra support to maintain airway.
_____ Assist MDs in maintaining airway until respiratory therapy arrives to take over.
_____ Prepare patient for transfer to operating room.

G. Debriefing Guidelines

1. What went well?
2. What could have been done differently?
3. Was everything done in the proper order for the patient?
4. Were all necessary supplies available and easily obtained?
5. Did the proper people respond?
6. What if the pediatric surgery team was paged and did not respond?
7. Were there any other interventions that needed to be completed by the nurse before summoning the MD to the bedside?
8. Were results of patient tests/labs missing that would have been helpful for background information?
9. How could this scenario be improved for the next time?

H. Suggestions/Key Features to Replicate or Improve

Prior to implementing a simulated experience, a key factor is to ensure that all participants must take the scenario seriously and perform assessments and treatments as if the patient were real. It was helpful for the nurse to arrive first on the scene and to receive a brief history from the handler before beginning the assessment. The collaborative approach between the nurse and the physician proved to be more realistic when assisting the patient. In the future, videotaping the scenario for a more interactive debriefing may be helpful.

I. Recommendations for Further Use

Rotating between different scenarios in order to keep the simulation novel may be prudent in the future. Ensuring adequate staff is available to participate in scenarios will maximize effectiveness and is essential. In addition, the use of either a high-fidelity or minimum-fidelity HPS would allow the handler to program vital sign changes, which would further assist in keeping the experience as realistic as possible.

It was noted during the initial scenario that there was no code button present in the treatment room, nor was there an available IV pump. This would have been unacceptable had this been a real emergency. As a result of this scenario, a code button was installed in the treatment room, and an IV pump was set aside for emergency use only. Each scenario proves to be beneficial in many ways, from improving the fluidity of emergency run situations to discovering essential equipment that needs to be on hand at all times.

J. Discussion of Simulation-Based Pedagogy and How This New Technology Has Contributed to Improved Student Outcomes

Emergency scenarios conducted on a regular basis will continue to increase confidence and decrease anxiety among staff, ultimately improving patient outcomes in urgent situations. This simulation has provided nursing staff the opportunity to practice their decision-making, problem-solving, and team member skills in a nonthreatening environment, which is a result that has been confirmed in simulation pedagogy (Day, 2007; Jeffries, 2008).

The above scenario has allowed staff to work through an emergency situation and to critically think through the process without an actual patient in distress. Simulations have been proven to be valuable learning experiences for the development of critical thinking skills, as supported by Childs and Sepples (2006). Additionally, debriefing after the simulation allowed for self-critique of interventions and reflection on improvement for future situations (Holtschneider, 2007). All participants were able to identify things in the emergency situation that could obstruct flow and fluidity of effective patient care. Making improvements on the unit following this trial emergency situation was an unanticipated positive outcome for all staff (noting code button and lack of IV pump). Preventing potential harm or delay in a child's emergency situation is an important outcome for all staff and supports the need for future simulations.

References

Childs, J. C., & Sepples, S. (2006). Clinical teaching by simulation: Lessons learned from a complex patient care scenario. *Nursing Education Perspectives, 27*(3), 154–158.

Day, L. (2007). Simulation and the teaching and learning of practice in critical care units. *American Journal of Critical Care, 16*(5), 504–508.

Holtschneider, M. E. (2007). Better communication, better care through high-fidelity simulation. *Nursing Management, 38*(5), 55–57.

Hunt, E., Walker, A., Shaffner, D., Miller, M., & Pronovost, P. (2008). Simulation of in-hospital pediatric medical emergencies and cardiopulmonary arrests: Highlighting the importance of the first 5 minutes. *Pediatrics, 121*(1), e34–e43.

Jeffries, P. R. (2008). Getting in S.T.E.P. with simulations: Simulations take educator preparation. *Nursing Education Perspectives, 29*(2), 70–74.

National Council of State Boards of Nursing. (2007). *NCLEX-RN examination: Test plan for the National Council Licensure Examination for Registered Nurses*. Retrieved June 18, 2008, from https://www.ncsbn.org/RN_Test_Plan_2007_Web.pdf

SBAR for students: Situation, background, assessment, and recommendation. (2007). *Nursing Education Perspectives, 28*(6), 306.

The SBAR technique: Improves communication, enhances patient safety. Situation-background-assessment-recommendation. (2005). *Joint Commission Perspectives on Patient Safety, 5*(2), 1–2.

Spunt, D., Foster, D., & Adams, K. (2004). Mock code: A clinical simulation module. *Nurse Educator, 29*(5), 192–194.

Recommended Reading

Maloney-Harmon, P., & Adams, P. (2001). Trauma. In M.A.Q. Curley & P. A. Maloney-Harmon (Eds.), *Critical care nursing of infants and children* (pp. 963–967). Philadelphia: W.B. Saunders.

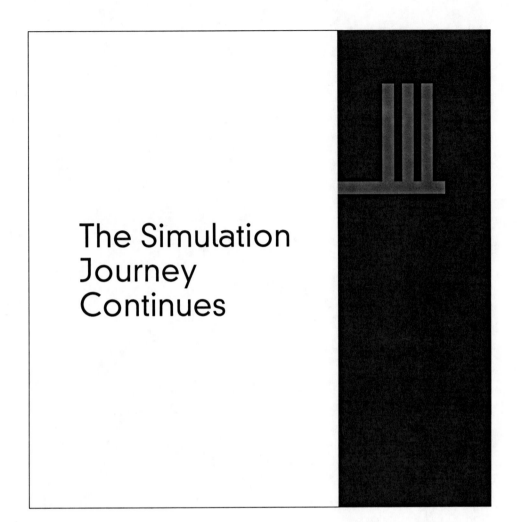

The Simulation
Journey
Continues

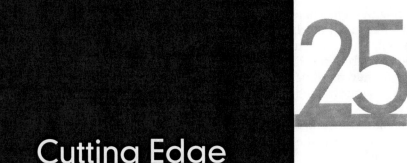

25

Cutting Edge Visions of the Future of Simulations

Philip A. Greiner, Suzanne Hetzel Campbell, and Chad M. Carson

Organizations, including academic institutions, have difficulty making change. New ideas often filter through layers of administration, dying along the way (Lencioni, 2007). This chapter discusses one experience where innovation was embraced and encouraged. Our experience may not work in other settings. However, it is important to dream and to think about opportunities that present themselves in our day-to-day work lives. It is in that spirit that we share this experience.

The opportunity stems from the current environment in which patient safety and outcomes are paramount. Studies from the Institute of Medicine, the American Association of Colleges of Nursing (AACN), and Quality and Safety Education for Nurses (QSEN) emphasize the importance of patient safety and quality of care in producing positive outcomes and saving health care organizations from financial burdens that result from hospital-acquired infections, falls, and so forth. Much of what is written about safety and quality care is focused on the delivery end. We realized that in order to provide the best education possible, the academic end had to begin incorporating patient safety and quality-of-care indicators into nursing education. At a recent presentation at Danbury Hospital in Danbury, Connecticut, Porter-O'Grady (2008) highlighted this point, recognizing the importance of the "frontline" for care delivery. The disconnect between education and clinical practice is emphasized when frontline nursing staff have not received sufficient information about patient safety and quality outcomes as part of their nursing education (Nursing Executive Center, 2008). The need for nursing education to embrace patient safety, quality outcomes, and technological innovation is paramount in order to bridge this gap, which leads to our story.

At an initial meeting with our corporate partner, the authors recognized the potential for the use of the Emergency Department software (Emergisoft*ED*) for academic applications. In particular, we recognized the potential to link simulation scenarios to the electronic medical record component in a way that enhanced the student's learning and experience. Further discussions of the identified potential for use in academic settings led to a site visit to see the software system in operation and to a broader realization of the potential that existed. After months of negotiations, Fairfield University and Emergisoft Corporation signed an agreement to explore the possibility of creating the product of our dreams.

Background and Significance

This agreement between an academic institution and a software company is based on the imperative within health care for an innovative approach to education for clinical practice. Specifically, the imperative stems from numerous Institute of Medicine (IOM) documents on patient safety, the need for technological sophistication and innovation in practice, and the integration of patient documentation with health care technology for quality improvement of health care services (Committee on Quality of Health Care in America, 2001; IOM, 2003, 2004; Kohn, Corrigan, & Donaldson, 1999). Additionally, the American Association of Colleges of Nursing (AACN, 2006) has published *Hallmarks of Quality and Patient Safety*, including recommendations for baccalaureate competencies to ensure high-quality and safe patient care. These competencies include components of critical thinking, communication, illness and disease management, ethical behavior, and information and health care technologies. The AACN competencies address health care systems and policies that contribute to safe and high-quality patient outcomes. The authors realized the transfer of technology from existing emergency department information system (EDIS) software to the integration of new software into clinical education and simulation directly addresses each of these competencies.

A group of studies from nursing (Cronenwett et al., 2007; Smith, Cronenwett, & Sherwood, 2007) examining the quality and safety of patient care by nurses recognizes the shifting role of nurses as leaders in documenting the patient's story and changing quality and safety in health care (Deese & Stein, 2004; Sherwood & Drenkard 2007; Weir, Hoffman, Nebeker, & Hurdle, 2005). These new roles and expectations for nurses require the use of information technology (IT), the development of leadership skills in patient safety, and increasing knowledge to drive a transformation of health care delivery. As Deese and Stein (2004) state, "It is nurses' interactions with information systems that in large part determine the efficacy of the system in promoting patient safety and improving outcomes" (p. 341). Innovative approaches to nursing education are required, including interprofessional education, enhanced communication, and the use of technology (Barnsteiner, Disch, Hall, Mayer, & Moore, 2007; Day & Smith, 2007).

More specific to nursing education, challenges exist in a number of areas, including finding sufficient clinical placements for the number of students, providing a breadth of experiences for every student, and assessing and evaluating student performance and documentation. In addition, accrediting organizations are asking for evidence of successful educational outcomes that are consistently measured and well documented (AACN, 2006). Current products on the market address one or two of these challenges, although not in an integrated and coherent way. A new approach to clinical education is needed that addresses these challenges.

One approach that has gained support is the use of simulations, primarily using human patient simulators (HPS), such as Laerdal's SimMan®. The simulation approach is earning a place in nursing education as a supplement to clinical practice with live patients. Increasing complexity in the health care environment and higher-acuity patients who are older and frailer mean that beginning nurses and students require a higher level of skills than ever before. As stated by Campbell (2007),

> *Simulation allows faculty members to take substance-specific information, such as a client's personal characteristics, health information, family components, and physical, mental, and emotional state and weave it into a real life scenario that enhances a students' comprehension of the material because it is meaningful. (p.124)*

Simulated patients allow for standardized learning experiences that can be viewed live by fellow students and/or recorded digitally for review and archival purposes. Simulations are being used to enhance learning, critical thinking, and practice with the goals of increasing patient safety, increasing efficient functioning, and introducing electronic medical record use.

The Fairfield University School of Nursing is taking a broader approach to simulation-focused learning that includes the use of case studies, role-play, low-technology HPS, high-fidelity HPS, and the inclusion of actors in simulated patient care situations as described in this book. This broader approach is unique and will provide superior, interactive learning experiences for students. Some limitations in using HPS stem from a need for faculty training, IT support, and development time to create the simulations.

The use of HPS opens up a variety of learning experiences for students to better prepare them for their clinical experiences and to provide faculty with a way to coordinate, assess, and record the mastery of specific competencies. One of the major gaps in this form of teaching is the nonintegration of electronic medical record keeping or documentation of the simulated events. In addition, because of institutional Health Insurance Portability and Accountability Act (HIPAA) regulations and the lack of a professional nursing license, students are often denied access to actual patient records and medication forms during their clinical experiences. The IOM reports that 44,000 to 98,000 deaths per year and in excess of $29 billion are linked to medication errors (Kohn et al., 1999). Research has examined adverse drug reactions (ADR), and specifically the role of the physician and nurse, and concluded that the use of electronic medical records decreased these ADRs (Deese & Stein, 2004; Morrison-Griffiths, Walley, Park, Breckenridge, & Pirmohamed, 2003; Simpson, 2001; Weir et al., 2005). With the existing gap between documentation and practice in both simulated and clinical experiences, nursing faculty are in a position to create a context within which to incorporate the use of electronic medical records for student information gathering on their patients as well as a system by which students can document their care. Running simulations in parallel with Emergisoft*ED* software and related products will help to fill these identified gaps. The new product line could wrap around existing HPS and simulation methods, thereby enhancing the experience of students and better preparing them to create longitudinal patient records and provide continuity of patient care. These records are also evidence of student competency for accreditation purposes.

Thus, the Fairfield University School of Nursing embarked on a more planned and comprehensive approach to nursing education and the use of simulation. The School of Nursing Advisory Board raised $1,060,000 to upgrade existing classrooms with state-of-the-art technology, including two simulation rooms hardwired to a control room and to two classrooms. In addition, this project supports faculty development, equipment purchases, and dissemination of our experiences on a regional and national level. Additional funding was secured from the Connecticut Health and Educational Facilities Authority (CHEFA, 2007) for the development of the Women's Health Simulation area. Partnerships with local agencies are being developed to explore expanded use of the simulation approach to learning with other health professionals and agencies. It is within this context that the initial meetings with Emergisoft Corporation took place.

The formal agreement between Fairfield University and Emergisoft Corporation was forged in recognition of the potential to develop a new product line that will address the challenges identified above. Given the present nursing shortage, retirement of clinically expert nurses, and increased acuity level of patients, patient safety and quality of care have come to the forefront as significant issues in health care and agency/hospital accreditation. Employers expect new graduates to work within a complex and high-acuity environment that relies increasingly on the use of technology. Society expects expert care and positive outcomes for every health care visit. This expectation creates a demand for providers who are well prepared and continually enhancing their professional development to include cutting-edge technology and evidence-based practice.

Emergisoft Corporation created its initial product, Emergisoft*ED,* to meet a recognized need for a best-of-breed EDIS to improve quality of care and increase patient throughput. Through collaboration and exploration with Fairfield University of the issues surrounding nursing education, Emergisoft Corporation recognized the need to create tools that will enhance classroom and clinical teaching without putting patients at risk. One current solution is the creation of simulated patient scenarios that expose students to critical patient events allowing students to develop advanced skills, including critical thinking, communication, delegation, and sociocultural awareness.

Goals of the Project

The partners recognized that maximum benefit could be achieved through the development of a new line of academic products derived from the best-of-breed EDIS product. The goals of the partnership are as follows:

- Create a dedicated, prepopulated database of patients blended with real-life experiences as a reference tool or basis for faculty to develop integrated scenarios for classroom and clinical instruction.
- Measure the feasibility for potential retooling of existing product components and features to create a system designed for academic applications.
- Integrate the use of components of the existing software with HPS in real-time scenarios.

Expectations and Conclusions

There are expectations of both partners in this collaboration. From the academic side, the expectations were threefold: (1) develop a new line of products that will enhance nursing education by making simulations easier to develop and run; (2) wrap these products around existing simulation methods so that documentation of care provided is an integral part of the scenarios; and (3) create an administrative structure through which virtual clinics and experiences related to management, leadership, and decision making can be organized. From the corporate side, the expectations were twofold: (1) develop a new product line that would expand the market presence of Emergisoft Corporation, and (2) recognize potential new revenue streams through the discovery of previously unexplored marketing and distribution techniques. Together, this partnership has the potential to create new markets for the product line linked to societal needs for quality care, technological sophistication, and a well-educated nursing workforce.

Health care educators need a variety of products to integrate simulation methods into their teaching. While HPS are a valuable tool, they are an incomplete answer to the simulation needs of most academic health care programs. Therefore, there is a need to explore and develop new products that augment, expand, and advance simulation use. This partnership is one example of an innovative approach to new product development. Corporations innovate by exploring new areas and new relationships. Partnerships with academic units provide a method for corporations to gain new ideas that can lead to new products and new markets. Together, the combined goals allow for a synergy that can benefit both organizations. The benefit to students at all levels is that their involvement in the process can result in an increase in both their clinical and organizational knowledge, better preparing them to join the workforce (Nursing Executive Center, 2008).

The process of developing the agreement between Fairfield University and Emergisoft Corporation has had positive repercussions for both organizations. Fairfield University was prompted to explore methods of handling profit-generating relationships so that funds were kept separate from the operating budget. They also had to develop documents related to intellectual property ownership and organizational ethics. Emergisoft Corporation has benefited from the creative thinking required in this partnership by exploring new approaches to sales and marketing and new methods of applying products in the training of hospital personnel. In addition, the innovative process involved in the development of this partnership has created an optimism that infuses the School of Nursing and has led to more active engagement with simulation writing and planning. In addition, exposure to a best-of-breed EDIS system has led to more active participation by faculty in the simulation process. As new products begin to be rolled out, the hope is that these will further stimulate faculty involvement and can be marketed to other academic programs across the country. Therefore, these products have the ability to increase the quality of simulation experiences for students, address the safety and quality demands of employers and patients, and decrease the scenario development time required of faculty.

References

American Association of Colleges of Nursing. (2006). Hallmarks of quality and patient safety recommended baccalaureate competencies and curricular guidelines to ensure high-quality and safe patient care. *Journal of Professional Nursing, 22,* 329–330.

Barnsteiner, J. H., Disch, J., Hall, L., Mayer, D., & Moore, S. (2007). Promoting interprofessional education. *Nursing Outlook, 55,* 144–150.

Campbell, S. H. (2007). Clinical simulation. In: K. B. Gaberson & M. H. Oermann (Eds), *Clinical teaching strategies in nursing* (2nd ed., pp. 123–140). New York: Springer Publishing Company.

Connecticut Health and Education Facilities Authority [CHEFA]. (2007). CHEFA grant for $99,999.00 women's health simulation expansion project. Pilot team: Suzanne Campbell (P.I.), Diana DeBartolomeo Mager (Co-P.I.), Phil Greiner, Sheila Grossman, and Alison Kris.

Committee on Quality of Health Care in America. (2001). *Crossing the quality chasm: A new health system for the 21st century,* Washington, DC: Institute of Medicine National Academy Press.

Cronenwett, L., Sherwood, G., Barnsteiner, J., Disch, J., Johnson, P., Mitchell, P., et al. (2007). Quality and safety education for nurses, *Nursing Outlook, 55,* 122–131.

Day, L., & Smith, E. (2007). Integrating quality and safety content into clinical teaching in the acute care setting. *Nursing Outlook, 55,* 138–143.

Deese, D., & Stein, M. (2004). Information systems and technology. The ultimate health care IT consumers: How nurses transform patient data into a powerful narrative of improved care [corrected] [published erratum appears in *NURS ECON* 2005 Jan-Feb;*23,* 45]. *Nursing Economic$, 22,* 336–341.

Institute of Medicine. (2003). *Health professions education: A bridge to quality.* Washington, DC: Institute of Medicine National Academy Press.

Institute of Medicine. (2004). *Keeping patients safe: Transforming the work environment of nurses.* Washington, DC: Institute of Medicine National Academy Press.

Kohn, L. T., Corrigan, J. M., & Donaldson, M. S. (1999). *To err is human: Building a safer health system.* Committee on Quality of Health Care in America. Washington, DC: Institute of Medicine National Academy Press.

Lencioni, P. (2007). *The three signs of a miserable job: A fable for managers (and their employees).* San Francisco, CA: Jossey-Bass.

Morrison-Griffiths, S., Walley, T. J., Park, B. K., Breckenridge, A. M., & Pirmohamed, M. (2003). Reporting of adverse drug reactions by nurses. *Lancet, 361*(9366), 1347–1348.

Nursing Executive Center (2008). Bridging the preparation-practice gap. Volume 1: Quantifying new graduate nurse improvement needs. Washington, DC: The Advisory Board Company.

Porter-O'Grady, T. (2008, May). *Advancing shared governance on the journey to excellence.* First Annual Spratt Distinguished Lecture series, Danbury Hospital, Danbury, CT.

Sherwood, G., & Drenkard, K. (2007). Quality and safety curricula in nursing education: Matching practice realities. *Nursing Outlook, 55,* 151–155.

Simpson, R. L. (2001). Information technology. Improve patient safety by leap(frog)s and bounds. *Nursing Management, 32*(9), 17–18.

Smith, E. L., Cronenwett, L., & Sherwood, G. (2007). Current assessments of quality and safety education in nursing. *Nursing Outlook, 55,* 132–137.

Weir, C., Hoffman, J., Nebeker, J. R., & Hurdle, J. F. (2005). Nurse's role in tracking adverse drug events: The impact of provider order entry. *Nursing Administration Quarterly, 29,* 39–44.

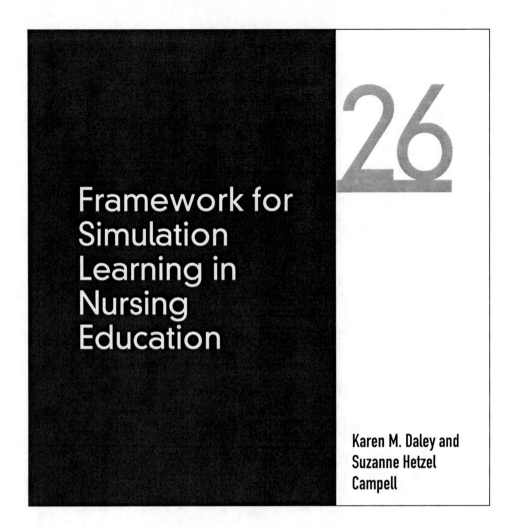

26

Framework for Simulation Learning in Nursing Education

Karen M. Daley and
Suzanne Hetzel
Campell

As stated early in the book, we believe a simulation-focused pedagogy of learning brings together an eclectic combination of learning, ecological, and nursing theory. As a result, we propose the following framework rooted in the current research on simulation, based on our experiences in teaching within a simulation-focused pedagogy, and combined with collective synthesis of the experiences of the contributors to this book. The following framework outlines the components underlying our perception of a framework of simulated learning for nursing education (Figure 26.1).

As stated in chapter 1, Jeffries and Rodgers (2007) have presented the Nursing Education Simulation Framework, which takes into account what is known about learning and cognition for the design of simulations (pp. 22–23). The Framework for Simulation Learning in Nursing Education presented in this text represents a student-focused approach to simulation-focused pedagogy for integration throughout the nursing curriculum. This learning takes into consideration the desired outcomes for nursing students and practitioners at varied levels. This framework presents an additional conceptualization of making simulation *real* for nursing education.

26.1

Framework for Simulation Learning in Nursing Education (Daley & Campbell, 2008)©

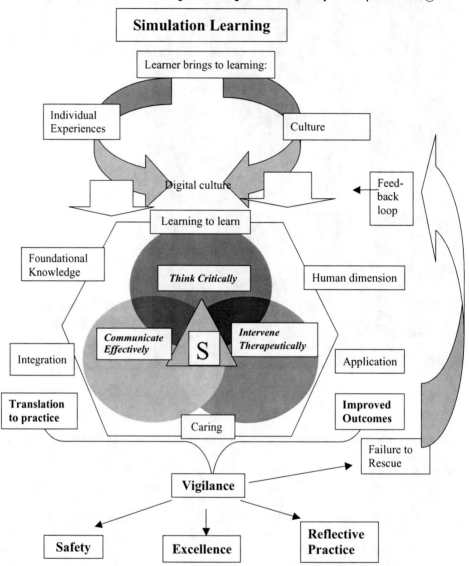

Guided by ecological theory, it is important to assess what the learner brings to learning (Stokols, 1996). Students come to the academic setting with a preset combination of individual experiences and culture as a lens through which learning experiences are viewed. Think, for example, how a nursing student approaches learning having cared for a dying family member as compared with a student without that experience. When considering a student's personal culture (including gender, age, and socioeconomic status) and the possibility of varied health belief customs, learning may be approached in a very different manner from that which faculty traditionally assumed. Students come to nursing from varied backgrounds (traditional undergraduate students, second-degree students, and adult learners) and cultural and life experiences, creating a challenge for educators to create a stimulating learning experience. In working with this diverse student population, one must take into account the digital culture in which they live and experience learning and move through it to reach a state of readiness for learning.

The central portion of the framework reflects the students' interaction with nursing education. Set within the context of any nursing program are often three broad goals and learning outcomes: Think critically, communicate effectively, and intervene therapeutically. These learning outcomes are represented in Figure 26.1 by the three circles that are overlapped by the triangle, representing simulation. Simulation as a teaching tool meets all three broad goals integrating simulation throughout the curriculum.

Allowing students to practice in a simulated real-life situation (in real time) requires that they use critical-thinking and clinical-reasoning skills. Performing the scenarios in conjunction with classmates enhances their use of communication and delegation skills. Their interventions cause immediate responses in the patient, and the debriefing period allows for evaluation of whether those interventions were effective or therapeutic, which helps students become reflective practitioners. The power of simulation lies in its ability to target these learning outcomes in an engaging and interactive manner beyond the didactic approach, which leads to better outcomes and more sustainable learning.

The triangle shape itself in the framework in Figure 26.1 depicts the three fidelities discussed by Fritz, Gray, and Flanagan (2007) that contribute to making the simulation as realistic as possible: equipment fidelity, environmental fidelity, and psychological fidelity. These fidelities provide the foundation for suspension of reality that is crucial to the success of the simulation experience. Paramount to any simulation is the debriefing period in which reflection on action can take place in order to set the groundwork and over time reinforce the formation of a reflective practitioner (Tanner, 2006).

When teaching a student, it is important to consider, Fink's (2003) six dimensions: learning to learn, foundational knowledge, the human dimension, integration, application, and caring. Represented by the hexagon in the center of Figure 26.1, these dimensions provide a support structure around which simulations can be planned and carried out. Faculty will create better learning experiences, set the stage for increased transfer of knowledge, and enhance the interactive component of their teaching by considering these dimensions.

As students move through a curriculum combining simulation and these pedagogical principles, the ultimate product is a student who learns vigilance. As an aspect of the overall concept of surveillance, nursing has focused on vigilance because of literature on quality outcomes (Almerud, Alapack, Fridlund, & Ekebergh, 2007; Jacobs, Apatov, & Glei, 2007; Meyer & Lavin, 2005). Once mastered, vigilance results in improved safety, excellence in nursing care, and reflective practice that addresses the patient's needs holistically. In addition, it creates a reflective practitioner who strives for lifelong learning, personal improvement, and enhanced satisfaction with his or her career.

Considering the nursing shortage and issues of retention among nurses, modeling this critical thinking, clinical reasoning, and reflective practice to help students recognize their passion for nursing could have long-term effects. Mastering vigilance—recognizing when patients need immediate and effective intervention—takes time and practice. In those instances when vigilance is not mastered, simulation learning provides a safe feedback loop back through the learning experience, allowing the student (or practitioner) another chance at mastery. The overall process works toward translation of knowledge to practice and improved outcomes for the student and program, as represented at the bottom portion of Figure 26.1. In addition, the quality of practitioners is enhanced, which will translate to safer care as well as more satisfied, caring, and reflective practitioners who continue to have the ability to transform the profession of nursing. The framework brings together a caring person who through mastery of vigilance reflects the three outcomes of safety, excellence, and reflective practice. Safety represents overriding concern for positive outcomes related to nursing care (e.g., no falls, pressure ulcers, or infection). Excellence in nursing is based on standards of care, quality outcomes, and evidence-based practice. Finally, reflective practice supports our conception of the caring professional who uses critical thinking, clinical reasoning, clinical judgment, and reflective debriefing in his or her daily practice.

Conclusion

How far we have come in so little time! Challenges still exist, such as assessment, evaluation, and the wise use of resources for simulation-focused pedagogy. It is our hope that our work, the work of our contributors, and our proposed framework will assist in moving nurse educators along in their journey to integrate simulation throughout their nursing curriculum. Go forth and simulate! Faculty, students, administration, and, most importantly, our patients will reap the benefits! The depth, breadth, and value of this book is in the stories told, the ideas shared, and the variety of teaching scenarios now available to all.

References

Almerud, S., Alapack, R. J., Fridlund, B., & Ekebergh, M. (2007). Of vigilance and invisibility: Being a patient in a technologically intense environment. *Nursing in Critical Care, 12*(3), 151–158.

Daley, K., & Campbell, S.H. (2008). *Framework for simulation learning in nursing education.* Working paper Fairfield University School of Nursing, Fairfield, CT.

Fink, L. D. (2003). *Creating significant learning experiences: An integrated approach to designing college courses.* San Francisco, CA: Jossey-Bass.

Fritz, P. Z., Gray, T., & Flanagan, B. (2007). Review of manikin-based high-fidelity simulation in emergency medicine. *Emergency Medicine Australasia, 20*(1), 1–9.

Jacobs, J. L., Apatov, N., & Glei, M. (2007). Increasing vigilance on the medical/surgical floor to improve patient safety. *Journal of Advanced Nursing, 57*(5), 472–481.

Jeffries, P. R., & Rodgers, K. J. (2007). Theoretical framework for simulation design. In P. Jeffries (Ed.), *Simulation in nursing education* (pp. 21–33). New York: National League for Nurses.

Meyer, G., & Lavin, M. A. (2005). Vigilance: The essence of nursing. *Online Journal of Issues In Nursing, 10*(3), 38–51.

Stokols, D. (1996). Translating social ecological theory into guidelines for community health promotion. *American Journal of Health Promotion, 10*, 282–298.

Tanner, C. (2006). Thinking like a nurse: A research based model of clinical judgment in nursing. *Journal of Nursing Education, 45*(6), 204–211.

Index

Index